MIND DIET FOR BEGINNERS

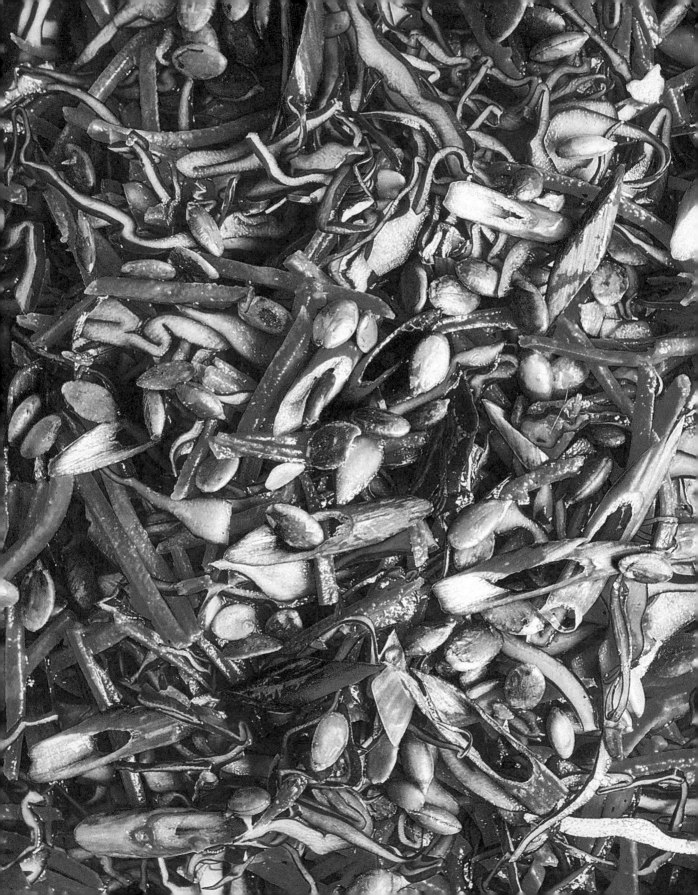

MIND DIET
for Beginners

85 Recipes and a 7-Day Kick-Start Plan to Boost Your Brain Health

Kelli McGrane, MS, RD

Photography by Hélène Dujardin

ROCKRIDGE PRESS

Interior and Cover Designer: Jami Spittler
Art Producer: Meg Baggott
Editor: Ada Fung and Claire Yee
Production Editor: Rachel Taenzler

Photography © 2020 Hélène Dujardin. Food styling by Anna Hampton.

Author photo courtesy of Kelli McGrane Nutrition LLC.

ISBN: Print 978-1-64739-818-7 | eBook 978-1-64739-493-6

R0

To my husband, Bryan McGrane.
Thank you for always being
my number-one supporter and recipe tester.

CONTENTS

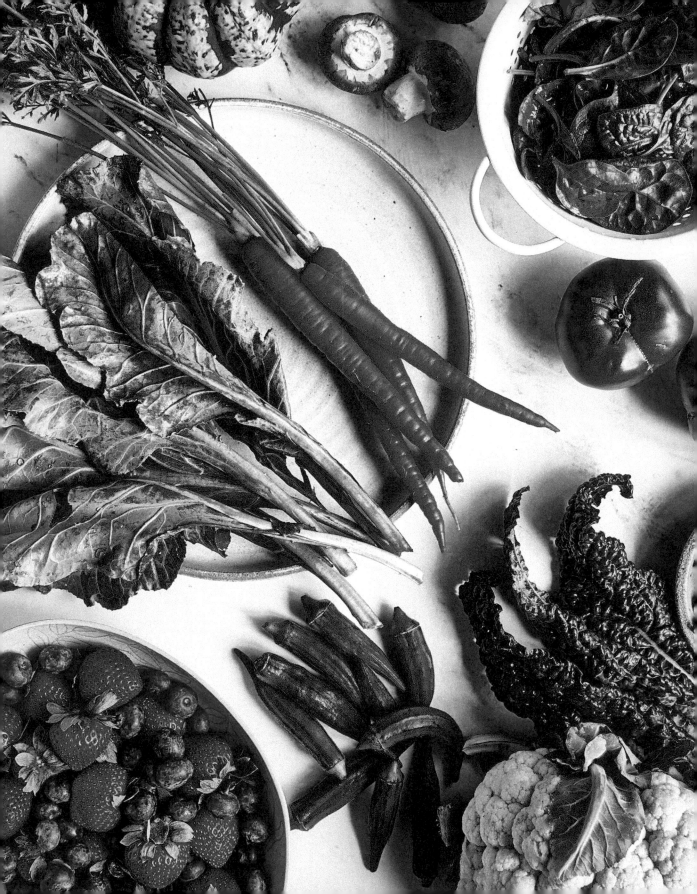

INTRODUCTION

For as long as I can remember, I've always loved two things: food and learning. Although I was instilled with a passion for eating and cooking at a young age, it wasn't until I was older that I became increasingly interested in how the foods we eat can affect all aspects of our mental and physical health.

Since becoming a registered dietitian and working in both nutrition research and counseling, I've gained an even deeper appreciation for how we can take control of our health by making more mindful food choices. Working with veterans at the VA, I had several patients who struggled with cognitive decline as they aged. Whether it was forgetting to take their nutritional supplements or not remembering how to prepare meals they used to make all the time, their gradual decline often meant that their nutrition suffered, as well. As their nutritional status worsened, I often noticed a further reduction in my patients' mental functioning. After working with these patients, I became an even bigger believer in maintaining a healthy diet and weight as we age.

Developed around nutrient-rich foods studied for their roles in brain health, the MIND diet can be an effective way to support a healthy brain and guard against cognitive decline as we age. With that in mind, in this book you'll find a clear explanation of what the MIND diet is and the science behind it, an easy-to-follow seven-day meal plan to help you get started, and simple, flavorful recipes to help you eat brain-healthy for the long term.

Whether you're caring for a family member who is suffering from brain disease or want to protect your own brain health, I wanted to create a resource to provide the knowledge and recipes you need to make a change and follow the MIND diet lifestyle. I hope you find it helpful!

PART ONE

MIND Diet 101

What we eat affects nearly every aspect of our well-being, including our brain health. The MIND diet was developed by scientists based on research showing the protective effects of certain foods on the brain. It encourages eating foods that have been linked to better brain health, such as leafy greens and berries, while limiting those that may negatively affect our brains, such as fried foods and sweets.

Part 1 of this book will provide you with information about the MIND diet, as well as practical tools and tips to get you started on your brain health journey.

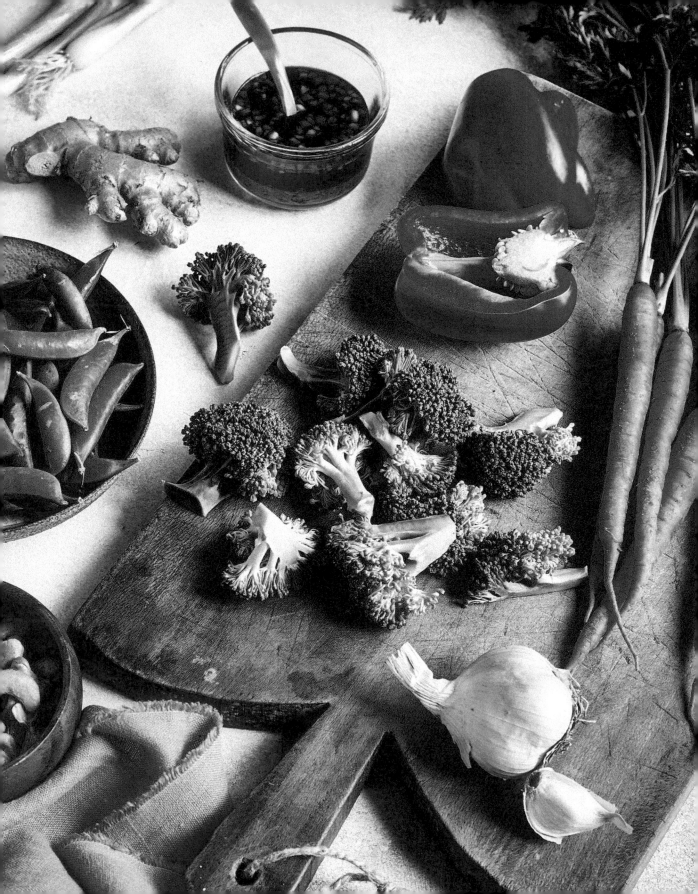

CHAPTER 1

Understanding the MIND Diet

Welcome to your MIND diet journey! Whether you've heard about the MIND diet before and are looking to learn more or are just reading about it for the first time, this chapter will give you the basics of what you need to know about the diet.

In this chapter, I will explain the research behind the MIND diet, help you understand the connection between diet and brain health, and give you guidance on which foods to include regularly in your diet, as well as which ones to limit.

What Is the MIND Diet?

Martha Clare Morris, ScD, and her team from Rush University Medical Center in Chicago developed a diet pattern based on previous research on the role diet plays in brain health, which was first published in September 2015 in *Alzheimer's & Dementia*. Now known as the MIND diet, this landmark study found that individuals with the highest MIND diet scores experienced a significantly slower decline in brain function over 4.7 years compared to those with the lowest MIND diet scores. In that same year, Morris and her team published a second study that found close adherence to the MIND diet was associated with a 52 percent reduced risk of developing Alzheimer's disease over 4.5 years.

MIND stands for Mediterranean-DASH Intervention for Neurodegenerative Delay. As you might be able to tell by the name, the diet is a combination of two well-known eating patterns: the Mediterranean diet and the DASH diet. The **Mediterranean diet** is inspired by the traditional eating habits of people in Mediterranean countries. It emphasizes eating healthy fats such as extra-virgin olive oil and nuts, fresh fruits and vegetables, and whole grains and legumes while limiting consumption of red meat and added sugars. Like the Mediterranean diet, the **DASH (Dietary Approaches to Stop Hypertension) diet** centers around fruits, vegetables, whole grains, and lean meats. Because it was developed to treat hypertension, it also limits daily sodium intake.

Both the Mediterranean and DASH diets have been linked to better brain health, so it's not surprising that the MIND diet borrows many of its guidelines from them. What makes the MIND diet unique is that it focuses on the specific foods and nutrients that have been shown to boost and protect brain health and reduce the risk of Alzheimer's disease and dementia.

For example, while the Mediterranean diet includes a general recommendation to eat more fruit, the MIND diet specifically recommends eating berries several times per week because research has shown a link between eating berries and having better cognitive function.

Although research on the MIND diet is ongoing, additional studies have already shown promising results. For example, a 2019 study of 1,220 adults found that higher compliance with the MIND diet was significantly associated with reduced odds of developing cognitive impairment over 12 years. Another study found a significantly reduced risk of developing, or a slower progression of, Parkinson's disease over 4.6 years.

As a registered dietitian and nutritionist with a passion for food and a background in research, I believe not only that the MIND diet is beneficial for brain health, but also that it can be a satisfyingly nutritious way to eat. My goal is to provide you with the information and recipes you need to follow the MIND diet.

Understanding Alzheimer's, Dementia, and Cognitive Decline

To discuss why the MIND diet is beneficial for brain health, it's important to first understand the differences between Alzheimer's disease, dementia, and cognitive decline.

ALZHEIMER'S DISEASE

Alzheimer's is an irreversible, progressive disease of the brain. The National Institute on Aging estimates that it affects more than 5 million people in the United States. One of the main features of Alzheimer's disease is the buildup of abnormal protein deposits that form plaque and tangles in the brain. There's also a loss of connection between nerve cells and, in advanced cases, even brain shrinkage. Symptoms include memory loss, confusion, disorientation, behavioral changes, difficulty speaking, apathy, and difficulty swallowing, especially later in the disease. Because Alzheimer's is a progressive disease, these symptoms often become more severe and noticeable as time goes on.

Currently, researchers are unsure of what causes Alzheimer's disease in most people. However, it's thought that it's likely a combination of factors, including genetics, environment, and lifestyle—including nutrition. Although there's still no cure for Alzheimer's disease, there is ongoing research on possible treatment and prevention strategies.

DEMENTIA

Unlike Alzheimer's, dementia isn't a specific disease but rather a set of symptoms that point to a decline in brain function, such as memory loss or difficulty concentrating. You can think of dementia as the umbrella that encompasses several disorders that cause chronic memory loss, including Alzheimer's. In fact, Alzheimer's is the most common form of dementia, accounting for 50 to 70 percent of dementia cases.

The second most common type of dementia is vascular dementia, which results from a lack of blood flow to the brain. It can develop slowly over time or suddenly, like after a stroke. Other forms of dementia include Lewy body dementia, Parkinson's disease, Creutzfeldt-Jakob disease, Wernicke-Korsakoff syndrome, and Huntington's disease. Other diseases, like HIV and multiple sclerosis, can cause dementia, especially in the later stages.

Although some types of dementia, such as dementia due to alcohol or drug abuse, may be reversible if treated early, most others—including vascular dementia, Alzheimer's disease, and Huntington's disease—result in an irreversible decline in mental function.

COGNITIVE DECLINE

Cognitive decline is a broad term for the reduction in baseline cognitive abilities. As you get older, you may notice subtle changes in your intelligence, memory, concentration, speaking, reasoning, and/or processing speed. For example, you may have difficulty recalling the name of a place you visited in the past. Although frustrating, with normal cognitive decline, the information isn't lost; it just may take longer for your brain to retrieve it.

The good news is that there are ways not only to reduce cognitive decline with age but also to sharpen these cognitive processes. Reducing stress, going for regular check-ups with your doctor, keeping your brain mentally stimulated, staying physically active, and eating a diet rich in antioxidants and healthy fats will all help keep your brain in top shape.

Assessing the Risk Factors

Other than aging, which is considered the strongest risk factor for cognitive decline and dementia, here are four of the top risk factors.

Family history. Individuals with a family history of Alzheimer's disease are at an increased risk for developing it. Although you can't change your genes, you can reduce your risk by making lifestyle changes and managing other health conditions.

Heart disease. Heart disease, as well as high blood pressure and high cholesterol, reduces blood flow to the brain, leading to nerve cell damage, brain dysfunction, and cognitive decline. Luckily, you can improve your heart health by exercising regularly, eating a balanced diet, maintaining a healthy weight, and not smoking.

Head injury. Recent research has found traumatic brain injury to be a key risk factor for Alzheimer's and dementia, as brain injuries can lead to permanent damage or death of brain cells. Accidents may not be able to be avoided, but you can reduce your overall risk or the severity of a brain injury by wearing a helmet when participating in sports, buckling your seatbelt, and "fall-proofing" your home.

Smoking and excessive alcohol intake. Both have been linked to an increased risk for cognitive decline and dementia. To reduce your risk, avoid smoking altogether and drink in moderation.

The Mind-Diet Connection

Your brain is your body's control center: It's in charge of your thoughts, senses, breathing, heartbeat, and movements. Your brain is working 24/7 to keep your body functioning efficiently, and it needs fuel to do so. The kind of fuel you give your brain will affect how well it works.

When you eat a diet of mostly whole foods that are rich in vitamins, minerals, and healthy fats, you're providing your brain with the nutrients it needs to perform its essential functions. For example, omega-3 fatty acids, healthy fats found in fish, can help build and repair brain cells. Antioxidant-rich foods like berries are also incredibly important, as antioxidants protect brain cells from inflammation and oxidative damage caused by free radicals (unstable atoms that can damage cells).

However, other foods have been shown to promote inflammation and stress in the brain. In particular, saturated fat, refined sugars, and ultra-processed foods have been shown to increase the risk for Alzheimer's.

Sugar and ultra-processed foods have also been shown to negatively affect your gut health. But what does this have to do with your brain? In addition to helping you digest and absorb nutrients from your food, the gut also plays an important role in regulating mood. In fact, about 90 percent of your serotonin (a hormone that helps regulate sleep, appetite, and mood) is produced in your gastrointestinal (GI) tract. The production of serotonin and other important hormones is influenced by the presence of good bacteria in your gut. A varied diet that's rich in fiber and low in refined sugars and ultra-processed foods supports the growth of beneficial bacteria.

Nutrients Your Brain Needs to Function

While an overall healthy diet is important for brain health, the following are the nutrients that are essential for proper brain function.

Omega-3 fatty acids. Omega-3 fatty acids are a type of fat that the body can't make on its own; we can only get them from our diet. Omega-3s are important for brain health because they strengthen the structure of brain cells. These healthy fats also improve blood flow in the brain and reduce overall inflammation. Good sources of omega-3s include oily fish, like salmon, tuna, mackerel, or sardines; walnuts; flaxseed; and chia seeds.

Choline. Choline is an essential nutrient that's required to produce a chemical called acetylcholine, which plays a major role in regulating memory, mood, and cognitive performance. Choline is also needed to synthesize DNA, which is needed for brain growth and functioning. Good sources of choline include eggs, chicken, shiitake mushrooms, and seafood like cod, salmon, shrimp, and scallops.

Flavonoids. Flavonoids are a large family of plant compounds that help protect brain cells against inflammation and oxidative stress. They've also been shown to improve blood flow and encourage cell and blood vessel growth in parts of the brain that are involved in memory and learning. In general, brightly colored fruits and vegetables, such as berries, grapefruit, and bell peppers, are good sources of flavonoids. Other sources of flavonoids include tea, red wine, and dark chocolate.

Vitamin E. Vitamin E is a vitamin that also acts as an antioxidant, which means it helps protect brain cells against oxidative stress and inflammation. Observational studies have shown an association between inadequate vitamin E and reduced cognitive performance, especially in older adults. Studies have also found a link between high vitamin E levels and a reduced risk of developing Alzheimer's. Good sources of vitamin E include nuts and seeds, natural peanut butter, leafy green vegetables, avocados, and trout.

B vitamins. B vitamins—in particular B_{12}, B_6, and folate—are important for brain health because they help produce the energy needed to develop new brain cells. Research has also shown that these vitamins help break down an amino acid called homocysteine. This is important because high levels of homocysteine have been associated with an increased risk for dementia and Alzheimer's disease. Good sources of these B vitamins include eggs, leafy green vegetables, whole grains, legumes, chicken, turkey, and low-fat yogurt.

MIND Diet Guidelines

Now that you have a better understanding of the connection between diet and brain health, let's get to the nuts and bolts of the MIND diet itself.

MIND SUPERFOODS TO ENJOY FREQUENTLY

On the MIND diet, there are certain foods, which I call MIND superfoods, that you should eat several times a week or even several times a day. These include the following:

Green Leafy Vegetables
Examples: Spinach, kale, collard greens, mustard greens, Swiss chard, arugula, microgreens, romaine lettuce, endive, bok choy, watercress, turnip greens

Recommended amount: At least 6 servings per week
One serving: 2 cups raw or 1 cup cooked

Other Veggies
Examples: Broccoli, cauliflower, zucchini, carrots, peppers, mushrooms, okra, eggplant, celery, cucumbers, pumpkin, tomatoes, sweet potatoes, winter squash
Recommended amount: At least 1 serving per day
One serving: 1 cup raw or cooked

Nuts and Seeds
For the healthiest option, choose plain raw or roasted nuts rather than salted or candied nuts.
Examples: Almonds, walnuts, cashews, pistachios, hazelnuts, pecans, chia seeds, flaxseed, pumpkin seeds, natural nut and seed butters; although technically a legume, peanuts are also included in the recommendations for nuts
Recommended amount: At least 5 servings per week
One serving: 1 ounce nuts or seeds or 2 tablespoons nut or seed butter

Beans and Legumes
Examples: Black, pinto, kidney, great northern, chickpeas, lentils, whole soybeans (such as edamame)
Recommended amount: At least 3 servings per week
One serving: ½ cup cooked (or canned)

Whole Grains
Examples: Brown rice, quinoa, farro, freekeh, wild rice, oatmeal, buckwheat, amaranth, barley, whole-grain pasta, whole-grain bread
Recommended amount: At least 3 servings per day
One serving: ½ cup cooked whole grains, 1 cup cooked whole-grain pasta, or 1 slice whole-grain bread

Extra-Virgin Olive Oil
The MIND diet recommends using extra-virgin olive oil as your primary cooking oil. It's high in anti-inflammatory monounsaturated fatty acids and contains protective antioxidants.

What About Drinks?

Staying hydrated is important for overall heath, so make sure to drink plenty of water. Tea and coffee contain flavonoids, so they are fine to have in moderate amounts as long as you limit the amount of sugar and cream you use.

Limit or avoid sweetened beverages such as soda, sweet tea, sweetened fruit juice, and sports drinks, as consuming large quantities of added sugars has been linked with diminished cognitive function and inflammation.

As for alcohol, the MIND diet recommends consuming up to 5 ounces of wine (one small glass) a day, due to its flavonoid content. Instead of wine, you could have 1 ounce of liquor or 12 ounces of beer, but you'll want to stay away from sweet mixed drinks, like margaritas.

MIND FOODS TO EAT REGULARLY

In addition to the MIND superfoods, you should also eat the following foods every week.

Berries
Examples: Blackberries, blueberries, strawberries, raspberries
Recommended amount: At least 2 servings per week
One serving: 1 cup berries

Poultry
Examples: Chicken and turkey
Recommended amount: At least 2 servings per week
One serving: 3 ounces cooked poultry, or a piece about the size of a deck of cards

Fish

Examples: Salmon, tuna, trout, halibut, cod, sardines, mackerel

Recommended amount: At least 1 serving per week

One serving: 3 ounces cooked fish, or a piece about the size of a deck of cards

Eggs

Eggs aren't specifically included in the MIND diet guidelines. However, eggs are a rich source of choline and B vitamins, and recent studies have shown a link between moderate egg intake and healthy cognitive functioning.

Recommended amount: No more than 4 servings per week

One serving: 1 large egg

What About Low-Fat Dairy and Sugar Substitutes?

Except for cheese, the MIND diet doesn't explicitly include dairy recommendations. However, I recommend consuming 1 to 3 servings of low-fat, unsweetened milk, yogurt, or kefir every day. Milk is an excellent source of calcium and vitamin D, and yogurt and kefir are rich in gut-friendly probiotics. If you are lactose-intolerant or have a dairy allergy, enjoy dairy-free alternatives such as unsweetened oat milk or soy milk instead.

Research is mixed on whether artificial sweeteners negatively affect gut health and increase your risk for dementia. Stevia, although a natural sugar substitute, also potentially has a negative effect on gut bacteria. Although small amounts are likely fine, it's best to limit your intake of sugar substitutes, just to be safe.

FOODS TO LIMIT AND AVOID

A healthy diet should be both enjoyable and sustainable. Therefore, while the following foods should be limited to maximize brain health, you can still enjoy them on occasion.

Red Meat

When eating red meat, choose unprocessed rather than processed meats, like hot dogs, sausages, and bacon.

Examples: Steak, ground beef, pork, lamb, bison, elk, other game meats

Recommended amount: No more than 4 servings per week

One serving: 3 ounces cooked red meat, or a piece about the size of a deck of cards

Butter and Margarine

Recommended amount: No more than 1 tablespoon per day of either stick or tub form

Cheese

Examples: Cheddar, mozzarella, Gouda, feta, Brie, pepper Jack, Parmesan, ricotta

Recommended amount: No more than one serving per week

One serving: 1 ounce of cheese or 2 tablespoons of shredded cheese

Sweets

Examples: Cakes, brownies, ice cream, pastries, cookies

Recommended amount: Fewer than 5 servings per week

One serving: ½ cup ice cream, 1 (3-inch) square piece of cake or brownie, 2 small cookies, or 1 small pastry

Fried and Fast Foods

Examples: French fries, chicken nuggets, fried chicken, fried fish, hamburgers

Recommended amount: No more than 1 serving per week

One serving: 4 chicken nuggets, 1 (4-ounce) piece of fried chicken or fried fish, 1 small hamburger (¼-pound patty), or 12 to 15 French fries

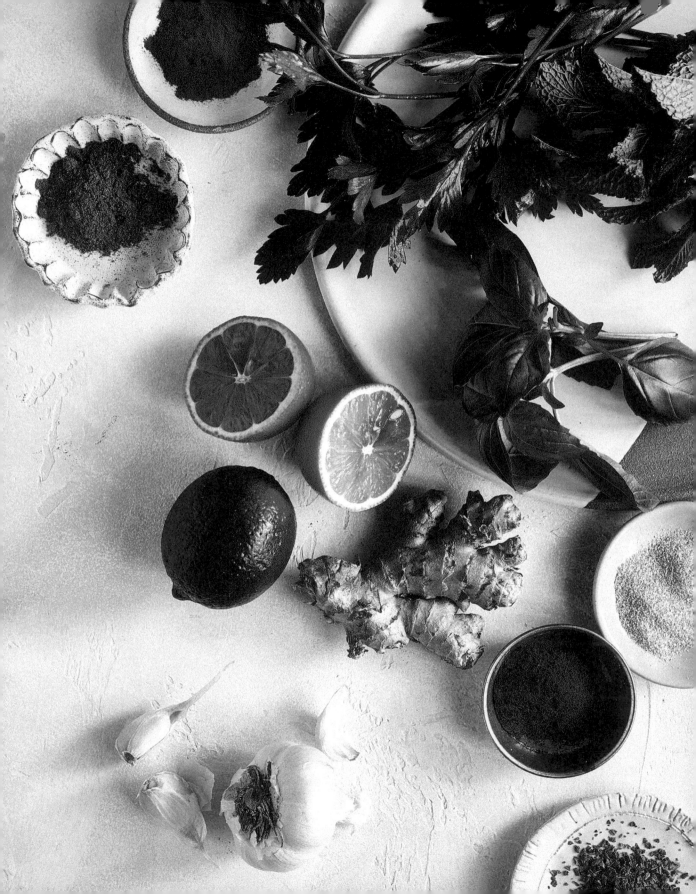

CHAPTER 2

Getting Started on the MIND Diet

Now that you know what the MIND diet is and the science behind it, it's time to talk about how to actually implement it.

In this chapter, you'll find all the information you need to be successful, including an easy five-step plan for getting started on the MIND diet, plus my top tips and tricks for making a lasting change to your lifestyle.

To make adjusting to the MIND diet even easier, you'll also find a 7-day meal plan, complete with a shopping list so that you can be sure you're getting started on the right track.

Step One: Set Yourself Up for Success

Unlike other diets you may have tried in the past, the MIND diet is designed to be a long-lasting lifestyle change to support and promote brain health throughout your life. As a result, while you don't need to totally restrict certain foods, it does require rethinking the types of foods you regularly have on hand.

As you transition to the MIND diet, you'll want to avoid keeping red meat, butter and margarine, cheese, sweets, and fast food at home. However, don't think that all your food has to go to waste. Instead, think about ways to donate or give your food away to families in your community. Homeless shelters, food banks, and local food rescue groups can all be good ways to give your food to those in need.

In addition to helping reduce temptation, getting rid of these foods is a helpful exercise for intention setting. As you're removing foods from your refrigerator and pantry, remind yourself that you're gaining better brain health and quality of life as you age.

Can't get rid of everything because other individuals in your household are eating those foods? You can still set yourself up for success by making MIND diet superfoods easily visible and keeping those other foods tucked away in the back of the refrigerator and the pantry.

Step Two: Go Grocery Shopping

It's also important to stock your pantry and refrigerator with foods to help keep you on track with your new lifestyle. Although you'll find a shopping list for the 7-day meal plan at the end of this chapter, here's a more general list of foods to keep on hand and put on your weekly grocery list. Stock up whenever they go on sale.

PANTRY AND COUNTER

- ► Avocados
- ► Canned fish such as salmon, tuna, and sardines: Look for ones packed in either olive oil or water.
- ► Extra-virgin olive oil
- ► Garlic
- ► Mixed nuts: Look for unsalted, either dry roasted or raw.
- ► Natural peanut or almond butter: Look for varieties without any added sugar or hydrogenated oils.
- ► Old-fashioned rolled oats: They're great for breakfast, as well as for making turkey meatballs and breading chicken.
- ► Onions
- ► Spices and dried herbs: Basil, cinnamon, chili powder, cumin, oregano, paprika, pepper, salt, and turmeric are good ones to keep on hand. Sodium-free seasoning mixes, like Italian seasoning, are great for adding quick flavor to your dishes.
- ► Whole grains such as brown rice, quinoa, and farro: I recommend keeping at least two types on hand for some variety in taste and texture.

REFRIGERATOR AND FREEZER

- ► Fresh and frozen berries
- ► Fresh and frozen leafy greens such as spinach, kale, collard greens, Swiss chard, and arugula
- ► Fresh and frozen vegetables such as broccoli, zucchini, bell peppers, cauliflower, Brussels sprouts, and frozen mixed vegetables
- ► Fresh, in-season fruits such as peaches, apples, cherries, and oranges
- ► Frozen fish fillets such as salmon, haddock, cod, and tuna
- ► Ground turkey: Look for at least 93% lean.
- ► Low-fat dairy milk or unsweetened nondairy milk
- ► Plain, low-fat Greek yogurt or unsweetened nondairy yogurt
- ► Skinless chicken breasts and thighs

Supermarket Smarts

Eating healthier doesn't have to be expensive and time-consuming! Here are some tips for saving time and money at the grocery store.

Buy in bulk. Buying MIND superfoods like grains, nuts, and seeds from the bulk bins or in larger packages will help you save money in the long run. The same goes for chicken. Simply freeze any raw chicken that you won't get to that week.

Buy in-season produce. Fruits and vegetables that are in season are not only cheaper, but they also often taste better.

Buy precut fresh vegetables. Although they may be slightly more expensive, buying precut vegetables will save you time when cooking. Plus, having precut raw vegetables on hand will make you more likely to snack on them instead of a less healthy alternative.

Don't forget about the frozen food aisle. Buying frozen poultry, fish fillets, fruits, and vegetables can often save you money, plus you don't have to worry about food going bad if you don't get to it that week. Using frozen produce also saves on prep time. Check the labels to make sure products don't have added fillers, sauces, or butter.

Step Three: Prepare Your Kitchen

In addition to stocking your kitchen with healthy foods, having the right cooking equipment and tools on hand will make it easier to maintain your new healthy lifestyle.

ESSENTIAL EQUIPMENT

4-quart pot with lid. This is great for making soups, sauces, whole grains, and pasta. If you plan on cooking larger batches, consider an 8-quart pot instead.

9-by-13-inch baking dish. I like glass or ceramic baking dishes for casseroles and other oven-baked dishes.

10-inch nonstick or stainless steel skillet. I like stainless steel because it won't chip, but it does tend to be a more expensive option.

Blender. Look for one with a motor that's powerful enough to handle crushing frozen fruits and pureeing soups.

Chef's knife. Look for a good-quality 8- to 12-inch knife that feels comfortable in your hand and has a full tang, meaning the blade is made from a single continuous piece of metal.

Cooking utensils. To cover all your bases, make sure you have a whisk, tongs, and a few spatulas and wooden spoons.

Cutting boards. For food safety purposes, it's best to have at least two cutting boards: one for raw meat, poultry, and seafood and another for produce. Wood, plastic, or bamboo are all good options.

Instant-read thermometer. To avoid the risk of under- or overcooking your poultry and fish, use a digital instant-read thermometer.

Measuring cups and spoons. Make sure you have measuring utensils for both dry and liquid ingredients.

Rimmed metal baking sheets. These are great for roasting vegetables and cooking sheet-pan meals.

NICE TOOLS TO HAVE

Cast-iron skillet. Compared to other types of skillets, cast-iron ones retain heat better, tend to last longer, and are more versatile because they're oven-safe.

Food processor. Buy one that comes with a shredding blade, which will save you time shredding vegetables like beets, cabbage, and carrots.

Salad spinner. To save space, look for a collapsible salad spinner.

Step Four: Live a MIND-ful Life

Much like the Mediterranean diet, the MIND diet is more than just what you eat. After all, diet is just one piece of the equation when it comes to brain health. In addition to incorporating more MIND diet superfoods, there are also lifestyle factors to consider for keeping your brain healthy and stimulated.

GET MOVING

As stated in the 2018 Physical Activity Guidelines for Americans, research has shown a strong association between increased physical activity and a reduced risk of developing dementia and Alzheimer's disease later in life, as well as general improvements in cognition.

Exercise helps reduce inflammation, increase chemicals in the brain that boost mood and processing, increase blood flow, and improve oxygen delivery to the brain. Oxygen delivery is particularly important, as increased oxygen promotes the production of neurons in parts of your brain that are in charge of memory and thinking.

The current recommendation is to engage in at least 150 minutes of moderate to intense physical activity each week. This can include brisk walking, running, hiking, swimming, skiing, biking, weightlifting, practicing power yoga, or any other activity that gets your heart rate up.

Not sure how to start? Try joining a walking group, taking a dance class, asking a friend to go on a hike, or signing up for an online workout class.

SLEEP WELL

While you're snoozing away, your brain is busy undergoing numerous processes that greatly affect your memory, capacity for learning, attention span, problem-solving ability, and creativity when you're awake.

For optimal health, it's recommended that adults get at least seven hours of sleep each night. If you have trouble falling asleep or staying asleep, make sure that you're sticking to a fairly consistent sleep schedule, avoiding stimulants (like caffeine) at least four hours before going to sleep, and turning off the TV or computer at least one hour before bed. Meditation, deep and rhythmic breathing, and reading are also good ways to calm your mind to help you fall asleep.

REDUCE STRESS AND THINK POSITIVE

We all get stressed out from time to time. However, studies have shown that chronic stress can lead to changes in brain structure, death of brain cells, shrinkage of the brain, and significant reductions in memory. So, to support your brain health, it's important to find ways to help manage stress levels and think positively.

How can you keep your stress levels down? Some research-backed ways to reduce stress include regularly exercising, socializing with friends and family, using essential oils, reducing caffeine intake, keeping a journal, listening to music, and practicing yoga or mediation.

PURSUE INTELLECTUALLY STIMULATING ACTIVITIES

Activities that keep your brain engaged and stimulated have been linked to improvements in memory and thinking skills. They may even help reduce plaque buildup in the brain. To keep your brain sharp, the next time you're bored, do a crossword or Sudoku puzzle, play a game of chess, or play a video game that involves multitasking and responding quickly to stimuli.

Be Kind to Yourself

Starting a new diet can be overwhelming and difficult. Whether you're caring for a family member with cognitive decline or are seeing signs of declining brain function in yourself, know that it's important to be kind and patient as you embark on this new health journey. Here are some self-care tips when you're starting a new diet.

Set realistic goals. Rather than striving to follow the diet perfectly, set goals that are realistic for your current lifestyle. Remember that you can always adjust your goals later as you progress.

Let go of guilt. Life happens. Just because you went off the diet doesn't mean you failed. Instead of indulging in negative thoughts, give yourself permission to let go of the guilt and get back on track.

Celebrate small achievements. Whether you completed the 7-day MIND diet meal plan or cooked a recipe from this book rather than ordering takeout, make sure to acknowledge and celebrate the small steps you're making on your journey to better health.

Step Five: Plan and Cook Healthy MIND Meals

One of the best ways to stick with a new way of eating is to plan your meals. Not only does planning your meals for the week help you stay on track, but it can also save you time, money, and energy.

Making a meal plan and shopping list over the weekend means you'll only have to go to the store once a week instead of running back to get ingredients several times. Meal planning allows you to choose meals that use similar ingredients, ideally ones you already have on hand. This saves you money on groceries and can help reduce food waste. Plus, when you have all your meals planned and groceries stocked at home, you won't be tempted to spend money on takeout.

You'll eventually find your own rhythm when it comes to planning meals for the week, but here are some steps to get you started.

1. **Figure out how many meals and portions you need for the week.** Will you be going out to dinner to celebrate a special occasion? Or going to a friend's house for dinner? Depending on what your week looks like, the amount of food you need to buy and prep will vary.

2. **Choose your recipes.** Take inventory of ingredients you already have and use that as a starting point for picking recipes. This is a great way to avoid food waste and keep your grocery list short. Another option is to pick recipes that use some of the same ingredients. In addition to this cookbook, it's helpful to have a list of recipe ideas and old favorites in a notebook or on your phone. That way, you know where to turn when you're short on inspiration.

3. **Write out your menu and grocery list.** It can help to write out your menu on a weekly calendar so that you know when you're making what. Once you have your menu written down, you'll want to make your shopping list. I recommend grouping ingredients based on where you'll find them in the store to make shopping even easier.

Ready to see meal planning in action? The next section is a 7-day MIND diet meal plan to help put these principles into action.

7-Day MIND Diet Starter Plan

Welcome to the first week of your new lifestyle! This 7-day meal plan will help you make the transition to your new, brain-healthy diet. In this section, you'll find the tools you need to be successful: a menu with a week's worth of delicious MIND diet recipes and an organized grocery list.

ABOUT THE PLAN

This 7-day MIND diet meal plan was designed with beginners in mind. To help cut down on the amount of food you need to buy and prep, the menu includes leftovers for some lunches and several recipes that use the same ingredients.

When looking at the menu, you'll notice that some dishes have asterisks next to them. These are the meals that you'll be making a double batch for and eating again as leftovers. The plan is designed for a family of four, so you'll need to make more if you're cooking for a bigger group or want more leftovers. Or if you're cooking for only one or two, you can either reduce the number of meals and eat more leftovers or freeze the leftovers to eat later in the month.

To make your week even easier, you'll find that none of the weekday breakfasts and lunches requires any cooking. Instead, they consist of a mix of leftovers, simple food pairings, smoothies, salads, and sandwiches.

Of course, if there's something in the meal plan you just don't like, feel free to swap in other recipes from part 2 of this cookbook, but keep in mind that you'll need to adjust the shopping list accordingly.

One final note: The shopping list only includes ingredients you'll need for breakfasts, lunches, and dinners. As a result, you'll need to add any snack or dessert foods that you'll want this week before you go shopping.

SHOPPING LIST

Produce
- Apples (2)
- Avocado (1)
- Bananas (3)
- Bell peppers (6)
- Berries, any kind (1 pint)
- Carrots, large (4)
- Celery stalks, large (2)
- Garlic (1 head)
- Kale, Tuscan (1 bunch)
- Lemons, medium (4)
- Limes (2)
- Onions, yellow, large (1), small (2)
- Shallot (1)
- Spinach, baby (20 ounces)
- Strawberries (1 pint)
- Sweet potatoes, medium (3)
- Tomatoes, cherry (1 pint)
- Zucchini, medium (4)

Dairy, Eggs, and Soy
- Eggs, large (13)
- Greek yogurt, plain low-fat (1 [32-ounce] container)
- Milk, low-fat or unsweetened plant-based alternative (1 quart)

Meat, Poultry, Fish
- Chicken, boneless, skinless breasts (2 pounds)
- Chicken, rotisserie (1)
- Salmon (4 [6-ounce] skin-on fillets)
- Turkey, 93-percent lean ground (2 pounds)

Frozen Foods
- Blueberries, frozen (2 cups)

Grains
- Elbow noodles, whole-wheat (1 [12-ounce] package)
- Oats, old-fashioned rolled (1 [42-ounce] container)
- Quinoa (2 [12-ounce] bags)
- Tortillas, small, corn or flour (24)
- Whole-grain sandwich bread (18 slices)
- Whole-wheat burger buns (12)

Canned and Bottled Items
- Beans, black (2 [15-ounce] cans)
- Beans, cannellini (2 [15-ounce] cans)
- Chicken broth, low-sodium (3 quarts)
- Chickpeas (2 [15-ounce] cans)
- Mustard, Dijon
- Soy sauce, low-sodium
- Tomatoes, fire-roasted diced (4 [14.5-ounce] cans)
- Tuna, albacore (12 [5-ounce] cans)
- Vegetable broth, low-sodium (40 ounces)

Seasonings and Oils
- Black pepper
- Cinnamon, ground
- Chili powder
- Cumin, ground
- Extra-virgin olive oil
- Garlic powder
- Ginger, ground
- Oregano, dried
- Paprika
- Red pepper flakes
- Rice vinegar
- Salt

Other
- Baking powder
- Baking soda
- Honey
- Mixed nuts (5.3 ounces)
- Natural peanut butter
- Nonstick cooking spray
- Vanilla extract

EASY SNACKING SUGGESTIONS

While this 7-day plan doesn't specify snacks or desserts, here are some easy MIND-friendly options to add to your menu.

- Fresh strawberries dipped in melted dark chocolate
- ½ cup of plain low-fat Greek yogurt mixed with 1 tablespoon of natural nut butter; add ½ banana on top
- Homemade trail mix with mixed nuts, dark chocolate chips, and dried blueberries or cranberries
- Hummus with whole-grain crackers and raw vegetables

Menu

	BREAKFAST	LUNCH	DINNER
MON	1 slice whole-grain toast with 1 to 2 tablespoons peanut butter and ½ sliced banana	Mayo-Less Apple Tuna Salad Sandwich* (page 92)	Slow-Cooker Turkey and Kale Minestrone Soup* (page 65)
TUES	Blueberry Muffin Smoothie (page 36)	Leftover Slow-Cooker Turkey and Kale Minestrone Soup	Black Bean–Sweet Potato Burgers* (page 82)
WED	1 cup low-fat Greek yogurt with ¼ cup berries and 2 tablespoons mixed nuts	Leftover Mayo-Less Apple Tuna Salad Sandwich	Lemon Grain Bowls with Cracked Freekeh and Roasted Chickpeas* (page 72), using quinoa instead of freekeh
THUR	1 slice whole-grain toast with ¼ large avocado and ¼ cup berries on the side	3 cups baby spinach, 3 ounces rotisserie chicken, ¼ cup sliced strawberries, and ¼ avocado tossed with Lemon-Dijon Dressing* (page 138)	Leftover Black Bean–Sweet Potato Burgers
FRI	1 cup low-fat Greek yogurt with ¼ cup berries and 2 tablespoons mixed nuts	Leftover Slow-Cooker Turkey and Kale Minestrone Soup	Leftover Lemon Grain Bowls with Quinoa and Roasted Chickpeas
SAT	Oatmeal Blender Pancakes (page 40)	3 cups baby spinach, 3 ounces rotisserie chicken, ¼ cup sliced strawberries, and ¼ avocado tossed with Lemon-Dijon Dressing (page 138)	Sheet-Pan Chicken Fajitas* (page 113)
SUN	Spinach and Sweet Potato Frittata (page 49)	Leftover Sheet-Pan Chicken Fajitas	Soy-Glazed Seared Salmon (page 93) with a side of quinoa

What's Next?

Congratulations on completing your first week of eating the MIND diet way! Now that you have a taste for what following the diet is like, let's talk about how to sustain your new lifestyle.

KEEP PLANNING MEALS

One of the best ways to maintain the MIND diet is by continuing to meal plan. Be sure to explore all the recipes in part 2 of this book to help you create your own menus each week. Refer to the meal planning tips in this chapter to make the process as easy and efficient as possible.

Also, don't forget that you also have a blank meal plan on page 147. You can make photocopies or download additional copies online at CallistoMediaBooks .com/minddietforbeginners.

USE A MIND DIET FOOD TRACKER

As you get more used to following the MIND diet, you may find that you don't need to meal plan to sustain your new habits or that detailed meal planning every week isn't realistic for your lifestyle.

Even if you don't follow a set meal plan, it can still be helpful to keep track of all the MIND diet foods you're eating each week and keep an eye on foods you may be eating too much of. The MIND Diet Food Tracker on page 148 is a chart that contains all the food groups mentioned in this chapter and how often each group can or should be eaten.

To use the chart, simply make a tally mark in the corresponding food group box each time you eat something during the day. Then, as you go through your week, you can quickly take a look to see whether you need to adjust your diet that week to stay on track. You can photocopy the tracker or download extra copies online at CallistoMediaBooks.com/minddietforbeginners.

ADVICE FOR LONG-TERM SUCCESS

The longer you stick with the MIND diet, the more you'll benefit from it. When you first start the diet, you may notice improvements in your energy and mood. You may even lose weight and improve your cholesterol levels. Over time, research shows that maintaining a MIND diet lifestyle can help protect your brain function as you age and reduce your risk of developing dementia and Alzheimer's disease.

When you first start a new way of eating, the excitement is often enough to keep you on track. But after some time has passed, motivation can start to decline. One way to stay focused is to keep reminders of why you started the MIND diet around you. Whether it's a picture of a loved one, a quotation, or a vision board, having a reminder somewhere easily visible can help keep that spark of motivation from going out.

Mindfulness is another tool for long-term success. Mindfulness means being present in the moment and making intentional decisions to honor your health.

It's also important to remember that a slipup from time to time isn't a failure and is actually very normal. When you fall off the wagon, simply acknowledge what happened, forgive yourself, and move on. If you're having trouble getting back on track, you can always hit refresh and revisit the 7-day meal plan in this chapter.

About the Recipes

All of the recipes in part 2 were designed to be easy for beginners on the diet to prepare. I hope you also find them enjoyable to eat!

EASY, BREEZY MEALS

Developed with beginners in mind, all the recipes in this book are either 30-minute, 5-ingredient, no-cook, or one-pot recipes. You can easily identify which type of "easy" each recipe is by looking for one of these labels at the top of the recipe page:

▸ **5-ingredient** recipes require only five ingredients to make (not counting salt, pepper, cooking oil, and water).

▸ **30-minute** recipes are those that take no more than 30 minutes to make, from prep to finished dish.

▸ **No-cook** recipes require no cooking at all.

▸ **One-pot/one-pan** recipes are cooked entirely in just one pot or pan.

HIGHLIGHTING THE MIND SUPERFOODS

All of the recipes also include at least one MIND diet superfood. These superfoods are bolded and in blue in the ingredient lists so that you can easily identify them and track all the goodness you're feeding your body and brain!

DIETARY LABELS AND RECIPE TIPS

Toward the top of each recipe, you'll also see vegan, vegetarian, dairy-free, and gluten-free labels to help you more easily find recipes that fit your dietary needs.

Each recipe also has one of the following tips:

▶ **Make It Easier** tips offer recommendations for how to make the dish faster, easier, or in a different way.

▶ **Swap It** tips provide substitutions for ingredients that may be difficult to find. These tips may also explain how to make the recipe vegan or allergen-friendly, or the tip may simply suggest ways to change up the flavor profile.

PART TWO

MIND Diet Recipes for Brain Health

Now that you have a solid understanding of what the MIND diet is, let's get cooking! In this part, you'll find MIND diet recipes to fit almost any mood or craving. From quick-and-easy Oatmeal Blender Pancakes (page 40) to impressive One-Pan Turmeric Chicken (page 116), my goal in developing these recipes was to highlight how you can follow the MIND diet while still enjoying variety and flavor in your meals. Whether you're new to cooking or short on time, all of the recipes you'll find are easy to make and don't require a trip to a specialty food store.

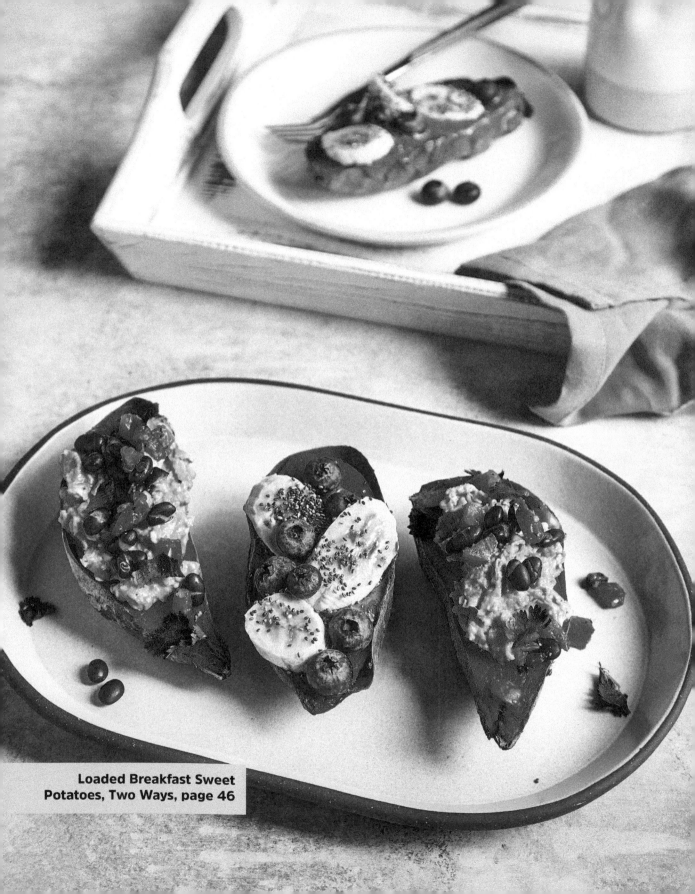

Loaded Breakfast Sweet
Potatoes, Two Ways, page 46

CHAPTER 3

Smoothies and Breakfasts

Raspberry-Lemon Smoothie

SERVES 2   **PREP TIME**: 5 minutes

30 MINUTES OR LESS | GLUTEN-FREE | NO-COOK | VEGETARIAN

This Raspberry-Lemon Smoothie is bursting with bright flavors—perfect for when you're in the mood for something light and refreshing. Although the low-fat milk and Greek yogurt both provide protein, feel free to add 1 tablespoon of almond butter or a scoop of protein powder for a filling boost.

1½ cups frozen raspberries

3 teaspoons freshly grated lemon zest

3 tablespoons freshly squeezed lemon juice

1½ cups low-fat milk or unsweetened milk alternative

1½ cups plain low-fat Greek yogurt

1 tablespoon honey, plus more as desired

Per serving: Calories: 276; Total fat: 4g; Saturated fat: 2g; Cholesterol: 19mg; Sodium: 145mg; Carbohydrates: 34g; Fiber: 3g; Sugar: 30g; Protein: 26g

1. In a high-powered blender, blend the raspberries, lemon zest, lemon juice, milk, yogurt, and honey on high until smooth and creamy.

2. Adjust the sweetness with additional honey as needed and pour into two glasses.

SWAP IT: For a creamier smoothie that's still naturally sweetened, replace the honey with 1 small frozen banana. You can also add spinach for a serving of leafy greens.

Energizing Matcha Smoothie

SERVES 2 **PREP TIME**: 5 minutes

5-INGREDIENT | **30 MINUTES OR LESS** | **DAIRY-FREE** | **GLUTEN-FREE**
NO-COOK | **VEGAN**

Matcha is a special type of green tea that's made by finely grinding green tea leaves into a powder. In addition to having an earthy flavor, matcha is a rich source of antioxidants and provides a boost of caffeine. When buying matcha, look for ceremonial grade for best quality and flavor.

2 cups fresh baby spinach

1½ cups unsweetened almond or soy milk

2 teaspoons matcha powder

2 small frozen bananas, sliced

1½ teaspoons vanilla extract

Per serving: Calories: 146; Total fat: 3g; Saturated fat: 0g; Cholesterol: 0mg; Sodium: 153mg; Carbohydrates: 27g; Fiber: 3g; Sugar: 13g; Protein: 4g

In a high-powered blender, blend the spinach, milk, matcha, bananas, and vanilla on high until smooth and creamy. Pour into two glasses.

SWAP IT: For a twist of flavor, swap out the vanilla extract for 1 (½-inch) piece of fresh ginger, use just 1 frozen banana, and add the segments from 2 small mandarin oranges.

Blueberry Muffin Smoothie

SERVES 2 **PREP TIME**: 5 minutes

30 MINUTES OR LESS | GLUTEN-FREE | NO-COOK | VEGETARIAN

This Blueberry Muffin Smoothie was inspired by one of my favorite coffee shop treats when I was growing up. I loved the contrast between the slightly tart blueberries and the sweet, cinnamon-speckled muffin base. Although texturally very different than a muffin, this smoothie has the same balance of flavors.

1½ cups low-fat milk or unsweetened almond milk

2 cups frozen blueberries

1 large frozen banana, sliced

½ cup old-fashioned rolled oats, gluten-free if needed

2 teaspoons vanilla extract

Dash cinnamon, plus more for topping

Per serving: Calories: 347; Total fat: 3g; Saturated fat: 1g; Cholesterol: 4mg; Sodium: 81mg; Carbohydrates: 70g; Fiber: 11g; Sugar: 38g; Protein: 11g

1. In a high-powered blender, blend the milk, blueberries, banana, oats, vanilla, and cinnamon on high until smooth and creamy.

2. Season with more cinnamon, if desired. Pour into two glasses.

SWAP IT: To increase the protein of this smoothie, swap out the frozen banana for ⅔ cup of plain low-fat Greek yogurt. If there's time, freezing the yogurt for 1 to 2 hours beforehand helps make the smoothie creamier.

Vanilla-Mint Green Smoothie

SERVES 2 **PREP TIME**: 10 minutes

30 MINUTES OR LESS | DAIRY-FREE | GLUTEN-FREE | NO-COOK | VEGAN

This smoothie is inspired by one of my favorite childhood treats: mint chip milkshakes. Instead of heavy cream and sugar, this recipe uses frozen banana slices, fresh avocado, and peppermint extract to replicate the vanilla-mint flavor and creamy texture. What results is a nutritious, naturally sweetened smoothie with a lusciously smooth consistency. Use even more mint extract if you like it very minty.

1 cup unsweetened almond milk or other milk alternative

2 cups fresh baby spinach

1 large frozen banana, sliced

½ small avocado, pitted and peeled

½ teaspoon vanilla extract

¼ teaspoon peppermint extract

Pinch salt

2 teaspoons raw cacao nibs or vegan mini chocolate chips, for garnish (optional)

Per serving: Calories: 160; Total fat: 8g; Saturated fat: 2g; Cholesterol: 0mg; Sodium: 190mg; Carbohydrates: 21g; Fiber: 5g; Sugar: 9g; Protein: 3g

1. In a high-powered blender, blend the almond milk and spinach on high until the spinach is fully broken down. There shouldn't be any small pieces left. Add the banana, avocado, vanilla, peppermint, and salt and blend on high until the mixture is smooth and creamy.

2. Pour into two glasses and sprinkle with the cacao nibs or chocolate chips (if using).

MAKE IT EASIER: To help blend frozen bananas, I recommend slicing them before freezing. Use frozen bananas within 3 months for the best flavor and texture.

Almond-Blueberry Overnight Oats

SERVES 2 **PREP TIME**: 5 minutes, plus overnight to chill

5-INGREDIENT | DAIRY-FREE | GLUTEN-FREE | NO-COOK | VEGAN

Overnight oats are an easy, filling breakfast you make the night before. I especially love this almond-blueberry version because it has a creamy, thick consistency and just a hint of sweetness. For more protein, feel free to stir in ¼ cup of plain Greek yogurt or dairy-free yogurt alternative to each jar of oats. I like to add a dash of cinnamon sometimes, too, for an extra kick of flavor.

1 cup old-fashioned rolled oats, gluten-free if needed

2 tablespoons chia seeds

1 cup unsweetened almond milk or any milk

2 tablespoons natural almond butter

½ cup blueberries, fresh or frozen

Per serving: Calories: 368; Total fat: 16g; Saturated fat: 2g; Cholesterol: 0mg; Sodium: 87mg; Carbohydrates: 47g; Fiber: 11g; Sugar: 5g; Protein: 13g

1. In each of two mason jars or other small containers with lids, add ½ cup of oats, 1 tablespoon of chia seeds, ½ cup of almond milk, 1 tablespoon of almond butter, and ¼ cup of blueberries. Using a butter knife, stir each jar of overnight oats well until fully combined.

2. Seal the jars and place them in the refrigerator overnight or for up to 5 days.

3. When you're ready to eat, spoon it up right from the jar. If the oats are too thick for your liking, add extra almond milk, 1 tablespoon at a time, until it reaches your desired consistency. You can also heat these oats in the microwave for 60 to 90 seconds for a warm breakfast.

MAKE IT EASIER: Overnight oats keep for up to 5 days in the refrigerator, so you can make your week even easier by making a week's worth of overnight oats on Sunday night.

Brain-Boosting Muesli

MAKES 4 cups   **PREP TIME**: 5 minutes

30 MINUTES OR LESS | DAIRY-FREE | GLUTEN-FREE | NO-COOK | VEGAN

Muesli is a Swiss breakfast food. Although it's similar to granola, muesli is often healthier because it's free of added sweeteners and oils. Plus, there's no cooking involved. Enjoy your muesli sprinkled over yogurt, in a bowl with cold or warm milk, or soaked overnight in milk or yogurt. For extra flavor, add fresh sliced fruit on top or a sprinkle of cinnamon. This muesli can be stored in an airtight container at room temperature for up to 1 month.

2 cups old-fashioned rolled oats, gluten-free if needed

½ cup toasted almonds or walnuts, or a mix of both

½ cup pumpkin seeds

1 tablespoon chia seeds

1 tablespoon ground flaxseed

½ cup unsweetened coconut flakes

½ cup dried cranberries or blueberries

Per serving (½ cup):
Calories: 258; Total fat: 13g; Saturated fat: 4g; Cholesterol: 0mg; Sodium: 4mg; Carbohydrates: 29g; Fiber: 6g; Sugar: 8g; Protein: 8g

In a large bowl, toss together the oats, almonds, pumpkin seeds, chia seeds, flaxseed, coconut flakes, and cranberries until well combined.

SWAP IT: The great thing about muesli is you can adjust the ingredients based on what you already have at home or find on sale at the grocery store. Can't find pumpkin seeds? Try sunflower seeds instead.

Oatmeal Blender Pancakes

SERVES 4 **PREP TIME**: 10 minutes / **COOK TIME**: 20 minutes

30 MINUTES OR LESS | GLUTEN-FREE | VEGETARIAN

These Oatmeal Blender Pancakes are a healthier way to enjoy a classic weekend breakfast. Made quickly in the blender, the pancakes have a soft, fluffy texture and just the right amount of sweetness. For a healthier option, serve them with a dollop of plain Greek yogurt and a spoonful of homemade Three-Ingredient Blueberry Chia Seed Jam (page 140) instead of traditional butter and maple syrup. Leftover pancakes can be stored in an airtight container in the refrigerator for up to 4 days, or you can freeze them for up to 3 to 4 months.

2 cups old-fashioned rolled oats, gluten-free if needed

1 small ripe banana

1 large egg

1 cup low-fat milk or unsweetened milk alternative

1 teaspoon vanilla extract

1 teaspoon baking power

½ teaspoon baking soda

¼ teaspoon salt

1 teaspoon cinnamon

Nonstick cooking spray, for greasing the pan

Fresh berries, for serving (optional)

Almond butter, for serving (optional)

1. In a high-powered blender, blend the oats on high until they have a flour-like consistency. Add the banana, egg, milk, vanilla, baking powder, baking soda, salt, and cinnamon and blend on high until well combined. You may need to stop occasionally to scrape down the sides of the blender with a rubber spatula. Let the batter rest for 5 minutes to thicken.

2. While the batter is resting, heat a large skillet or griddle pan over medium-low heat. Lightly grease it with nonstick cooking spray.

3. Pour ⅓ cup of batter per pancake into the heated pan. The pancakes are ready to flip when the bubbles that have formed on top start to pop and the edges look set, about 3 minutes. Using a spatula, flip each pancake and cook for another 1 to 2 minutes, or until the bottom is golden brown. Transfer the cooked pancakes to a plate and cover with foil to keep warm. Repeat with the remaining batter.

4. Serve pancakes topped with fresh berries and almond butter (if using) or your favorite toppings.

SWAP IT: To make this recipe vegan, use an unsweetened milk alternative, such as oat milk or almond milk, and swap out the egg for a flax egg. To make a flax egg, combine 1 tablespoon of ground flaxseed with 2½ tablespoons of water. Mix well, then let the mixture set for 5 minutes.

Toasted Almond–Quinoa Breakfast Bowl

SERVES 2 **PREP TIME**: 5 minutes / **COOK TIME**: 20 minutes

5-INGREDIENT | **30 MINUTES OR LESS** | **DAIRY-FREE** | **GLUTEN-FREE**
ONE-POT | **VEGAN**

This nutty quinoa breakfast bowl is a nutritious way to change up your normal breakfast routine. If you aren't a fan of the texture of oatmeal, you'll love the chewy and hearty texture of this bowl. Although I love the simple flavors of vanilla and almonds, you can make it even cozier by adding warmed frozen blueberries, a dash of cinnamon or cardamom, or a drizzle of maple syrup.

½ cup uncooked **quinoa, rinsed**

1 cup unsweetened **almond milk, plus more as needed**

⅛ teaspoon **salt**

½ teaspoon **vanilla extract**

¼ cup sliced **almonds, toasted**

Per serving: Calories: 535; Total fat: 24g; Saturated fat: 2g; Cholesterol: 0mg; Sodium: 470mg; Carbohydrates: 62g; Fiber: 9g; Sugar: 7g; Protein: 19g

1. Place a small saucepan over medium-high heat. Add the quinoa, almond milk, and salt. Bring to a low boil. When it's just boiling, reduce the heat to medium-low, cover, and simmer for 15 minutes. If it starts bubbling rather than gently simmering, reduce the heat to low.

2. After 15 minutes, remove the pan from the heat and let it rest for 5 minutes, or until the quinoa has absorbed all the liquid. Remove the lid and stir in the vanilla.

3. Evenly divide the quinoa between two bowls and top with the toasted almonds and any other toppings you like. For a thinner, more porridge-like consistency, stir in additional warm almond milk.

MAKE IT EASIER: This breakfast bowl can be made up to 4 days ahead of time. To reheat, simply place it in a microwave-safe bowl and add a splash of almond milk on top. Microwave for 30 to 60 seconds.

Slow-Cooker Cinnamon-Walnut Oatmeal

SERVES 6 **PREP TIME**: 5 minutes / **COOK TIME**: 7 to 8 hours on Low or 4 hours on High

GLUTEN-FREE | ONE-POT | VEGETARIAN

Set this to cook before you go to bed, and you'll wake up to a kitchen filled with the warming aromas of cinnamon, banana, and vanilla. Just make sure not to oversleep, as the oats may start to burn after 8 hours. Do not substitute quick-cooking, instant, or old-fashioned rolled oats for the steel-cut, as they'll become too mushy and may even burn in the slow cooker.

1½ cups steel-cut oats, gluten-free if needed

4 cups water

2 cups low-fat milk or unsweetened milk alternative

2 large ripe bananas, mashed

2 teaspoons vanilla extract

⅛ teaspoon salt

1½ teaspoons cinnamon

½ cup chopped walnuts, toasted

Sliced strawberries, for topping

Honey, for topping

Natural peanut butter, for topping

Per serving (excluding toppings): Calories: 289; Total fat: 9g; Saturated fat: 1g; Cholesterol: 2mg; Sodium: 87mg; Carbohydrates: 44g; Fiber: 6g; Sugar: 11g; Protein: 10g

1. In a 4- or 6-quart slow cooker, stir together the oats, water, milk, bananas, vanilla, salt, cinnamon, and walnuts until well combined. Cover and cook on low for 7 to 8 hours or on high for 4 hours.

2. Serve topped with more walnuts, strawberries, honey, and peanut butter or other toppings you like.

MAKE IT EASIER: Leftovers will keep in the refrigerator for up to 1 week, so make a big batch on the weekend and have breakfast at the ready for the rest of the week! To reheat, add 1 to 2 tablespoons of milk or water and warm in the microwave for 30 to 60 seconds.

Savory Steel-Cut Oats

SERVES 2 **PREP TIME**: 5 minutes / **COOK TIME**: 35 minutes

5-INGREDIENT | DAIRY-FREE | GLUTEN-FREE | VEGETARIAN

Oatmeal is a classic, healthy breakfast that's typically enjoyed sweet. This recipe is a savory twist; it's topped with an over-easy egg and fresh avocado slices for an indulgent flavor and texture. Feel free to bump up the nutrition even more by adding other vegetables, such as sautéed mushrooms or cooked spinach.

1½ cups water

Salt

½ cup steel-cut oats, gluten-free if needed

Nonstick cooking spray

2 large eggs

Freshly ground black pepper

½ large avocado, sliced

Low-sodium soy sauce, for topping (optional)

Red pepper flakes, for topping (optional)

Hot sauce, for topping (optional)

Per serving: Calories: 277; Total fat: 13g; Saturated fat: 3g; Cholesterol: 164mg; Sodium: 60mg; Carbohydrates: 31g; Fiber: 6g; Sugar: 1g; Protein: 12g

1. In a medium saucepan over high heat, bring the water and a pinch of salt to a boil. Add the steel-cut oats and boil for 1 minute. Then reduce the heat to medium-low and cover. Simmer for 20 to 30 minutes, or until the water has been absorbed and the oats are soft but chewy. Remove from the heat but keep the cover on.

2. Place a small skillet over medium-low heat and lightly grease it with cooking spray. One at a time, carefully crack each egg into a small bowl and then pour it into the center of the heated skillet. Lightly season the eggs with salt and pepper.

3. When the egg whites are just set, carefully flip them and cook for an additional 10 to 15 seconds. Remove the pan from the heat.

4. Divide the cooked oats between two bowls and top each with a cooked egg and half of the avocado slices. Top with a splash of soy sauce, red pepper flakes, or a dash of hot sauce (if using).

SWAP IT: If you don't like over-easy eggs, you can also serve them poached or soft-boiled. The key is having a runny yolk to coat the cooked oats as you eat them.

Smoked Salmon and Spinach Quinoa Bowl

SERVES 4 **PREP TIME**: 10 minutes / **COOK TIME**: 20 minutes

30 MINUTES OR LESS | GLUTEN-FREE

Smoked salmon is an easy, flavor-packed way to get some omega-3s in the morning. What's great about this recipe is it can be prepped ahead of time and is easily customizable based on what you have on hand. Feel free to use any whole grains that you have left over in your refrigerator. You can even use leftover potatoes, sweet potatoes, or butternut squash.

1 cup uncooked quinoa, rinsed

2 cups water

1 tablespoon extra-virgin olive oil

1 cup sliced mushrooms

⅛ teaspoon salt, plus more for seasoning

Freshly ground black pepper

4 cups fresh baby spinach

12 ounces smoked salmon

¼ cup plain low-fat Greek yogurt

2 teaspoons freshly squeezed lemon juice

1 tablespoon minced fresh dill, or 1 teaspoon dried

Per serving: Calories: 309; Total fat: 10g; Saturated fat: 2g; Cholesterol: 21mg; Sodium: 678mg; Carbohydrates: 30g; Fiber: 4g; Sugar: 4g; Protein: 25g

1. In a medium saucepan over high heat, add the quinoa and water and bring to a boil. Cover and reduce the heat to medium-low. Simmer for 15 minutes. Remove from the heat and let the quinoa sit for 5 minutes before fluffing with a fork.

2. While the quinoa cooks, in a medium skillet, heat the oil over medium-high heat. Add the mushrooms and season with a pinch of salt and pepper. Cook for 3 minutes, stir, and cook for another 2 minutes, or until softened. Add the spinach and cook for 2 to 3 minutes, or until it wilts. If you need a little extra steam, add 2 to 3 teaspoons of water. Season with salt and pepper and set aside.

3. Evenly divide the quinoa among four bowls and top with the sautéed vegetables and smoked salmon.

4. In a small bowl, whisk together the yogurt, lemon juice, salt, and dill. Drizzle over the bowls.

MAKE IT EASIER: Prepare the quinoa, vegetables, and yogurt dressing a day or two in advance. Then all you'll need to do in the morning is reheat the quinoa and vegetables and assemble your bowl.

Loaded Breakfast Sweet Potatoes, Two Ways

SERVES 2 **PREP TIME**: 10 minutes / **COOK TIME**: 15 minutes

5-INGREDIENT | 30 MINUTES OR LESS | DAIRY-FREE | GLUTEN-FREE
VEGETARIAN

Change up your usual breakfasts with these loaded sweet potatoes. Whether you want to bring out the sweetness with drippy peanut butter and sliced bananas or are more in the mood for a savory breakfast, this recipe provides you with two nutritious and filling options to choose from. This recipe is less specific and more of an idea, so feel free to mix and match ingredients and seasonings to create your ideal morning meal.

For sweet loaded sweet potatoes

2 small sweet potatoes

2 tablespoons almond butter or peanut butter

1 small banana, sliced

¼ cup blueberries

2 tablespoons chia seeds or hemp hearts

For savory loaded sweet potatoes

2 small sweet potatoes

Nonstick cooking spray

2 large eggs

¼ cup cooked or canned black beans

¼ cup salsa

Fresh cilantro leaves, for garnish (optional)

To make sweet loaded sweet potatoes

1. Using a fork, poke a few holes into each sweet potato, then place them on a microwave-safe plate. Microwave on high for 5 minutes. Then flip and microwave for another 5 to 7 minutes, or until you can easily pierce each sweet potato with a fork.

2. Slice the sweet potatoes in half and drizzle 1 tablespoon of almond or peanut butter over each. Top with banana slices, blueberries, and chia seeds or hemp hearts.

To make savory loaded sweet potatoes

3. Using a fork, poke a few holes into each sweet potato, then place the potatoes on a microwave-safe plate. Microwave on high for 5 minutes. Then flip and microwave for another 5 to 7 minutes, or until you can easily pierce each sweet potato with a fork.

Per serving (sweet):
Calories: 258; Total fat: 11g; Saturated fat: 2g; Cholesterol: 0mg; Sodium: 40mg; Carbohydrates: 36g; Fiber: 9g; Sugar: 12g; Protein: 7g

Per serving (savory):
Calories: 167; Total fat: 5g; Saturated fat: 2g; Cholesterol: 164mg; Sodium: 406mg; Carbohydrates: 22g; Fiber: 5g; Sugar: 5g; Protein: 9g

4. While the sweet potatoes are cooking, place a small skillet over medium-low heat and lightly grease it with nonstick cooking spray. In a small bowl, beat the eggs and pour them into the heated skillet. Using a heatproof spatula, move the eggs around in the pan to scramble them. Remove from the heat when they look set but not dry, 3 to 5 minutes.

5. Slice the sweet potatoes in half and place half of the scrambled eggs on top of each. Top with black beans, salsa, and cilantro (if using).

SWAP IT: If you prefer roasted sweet potatoes over microwaved ones, roast your sweet potatoes for 1 hour at 400°F a day or two ahead of time, then simply reheat one in the morning.

Green Shakshuka

SERVES 4 **PREP TIME**: 10 minutes / **COOK TIME**: 20 minutes

30 MINUTES OR LESS | DAIRY-FREE | GLUTEN-FREE | ONE-POT | VEGETARIAN

Shakshuka is a traditional Middle Eastern dish of eggs poached in a spiced tomato sauce. This dish takes flavor inspiration from the classic but replaces the tomato sauce with MIND diet superfoods: baby spinach, zucchini, and Brussels sprouts. This dish is perfect for brunch or dinner. I recommend serving this Green Shakshuka with a loaf of crusty whole-grain bread (or a gluten-free loaf, if needed).

2 tablespoons
extra-virgin olive oil

1 shallot, diced

2 garlic cloves, minced

½ pound Brussels
sprouts, shaved or sliced

1 medium
zucchini, grated

1 teaspoon ground cumin

½ teaspoon salt

¼ teaspoon freshly
ground black pepper

2 cups fresh
baby spinach

4 large eggs

1 tablespoon water

1 large avocado, diced

Per serving: Calories: 257; Total fat: 17g; Saturated fat: 3g; Cholesterol: 164mg; Sodium: 399mg; Carbohydrates: 18g; Fiber: 8g; Sugar: 5g; Protein: 12g

1. In a large skillet, heat the oil over medium heat. Add the shallot and cook for 2 minutes, or until it becomes soft and fragrant. Add the garlic and cook for another 30 seconds, or until fragrant.

2. Add the Brussels sprouts to the pan and cook for 5 minutes, or until soft, stirring frequently. Next, add the zucchini, cumin, salt, and pepper. Cook for 1 minute, then add the spinach. Cook for 2 to 3 minutes, or until the spinach just starts to wilt.

3. Reduce the heat to low. Using a spatula, create four small wells in the vegetable mixture. Crack an egg into a small bowl, then pour it into one of the wells. Repeat with the remaining eggs.

4. Add the water to the pan and cover. Steam for 3 to 5 minutes, or until the egg whites are set but the yolks are still runny.

5. Remove the pan from the heat and top with the diced avocado.

SWAP IT: Feel free to swap out any of the vegetables in this recipe with what you have in the refrigerator or what is in season. For example, kale, chopped bell peppers, diced jalapeño peppers, or sliced mushrooms would all work well.

Spinach and Sweet Potato Frittata

SERVES 6 **PREP TIME**: 10 minutes / **COOK TIME**: 30 minutes

GLUTEN-FREE | ONE-POT | VEGETARIAN

A frittata is a simple baked egg dish. Although typically made from eggs, milk, and cheese, to make it more MIND diet-friendly, this recipe leaves out the cheese and adds flavor and nutrition with sautéed spinach, sweet potato, and shallots. Although you can enjoy it on its own for a light meal, I recommend serving this veggie frittata with a side of whole-grain toast and some fresh berries.

1 tablespoon extra-virgin olive oil

1 medium sweet potato, peeled and cut into ½-inch cubes

1 shallot, diced

¼ teaspoon salt, plus more for seasoning

Freshly ground black pepper

3 cups roughly chopped fresh baby spinach

12 large eggs

½ cup low-fat milk or unsweetened milk alternative

½ teaspoon dried oregano

Per serving: Calories: 190; Total fat: 12g; Saturated fat: 3g; Cholesterol: 329mg; Sodium: 266mg; Carbohydrates: 8g; Fiber: 1g; Sugar: 4g; Protein: 13g

1. Preheat the oven to 350°F.

2. In a 12-inch oven-safe skillet, heat the oil over medium-high heat. Add the sweet potato and shallot and season with a pinch of salt and pepper. Cook for 4 minutes, or until the sweet potato has softened slightly. Add the spinach and cook for 1 minute, or until wilted. Reduce the heat to medium-low.

3. In a large bowl, whisk together the eggs, milk, salt, and oregano until well combined. Carefully pour the egg mixture into the pan with the vegetables and cook for 3 to 5 minutes, or until the sides of the eggs are set.

4. Turn off the stove and place the skillet on the middle rack in the oven. Bake for 20 minutes, or until the middle is set and no longer jiggles. Remove from the oven and cool for 2 to 3 minutes. Slice into 6 pieces to serve.

SWAP IT: If you don't have an oven-safe skillet, transfer the cooked vegetables into a lightly greased 9-by-13-inch pan. Pour the eggs into the pan and bake for 25 to 30 minutes.

Farmers' Market Tofu Scramble

SERVES 4 **PREP TIME**: 10 minutes / **COOK TIME**: 20 minutes

30 MINUTES OR LESS | DAIRY-FREE | GLUTEN-FREE | ONE-POT | VEGAN

Breakfast scrambles are the perfect way to enjoy seasonal produce, which is why this recipe doesn't list specific vegetables. Instead, use whatever is in season at your local farmers' market or supermarket. We're replacing scrambled eggs with crumbled tofu and a few simple seasonings for a delicious, protein-packed vegan alternative.

2 tablespoons
extra-virgin olive oil

2 cups diced mixed
vegetables

2 garlic cloves, minced

½ teaspoon salt, plus
more for seasoning

½ teaspoon freshly
ground black pepper,
plus more for seasoning

1 (14-ounce) package
firm tofu, drained and
patted dry

½ teaspoon ground
turmeric

2 tablespoons nutritional
yeast (optional)

2 cups chopped
leafy greens

Hot sauce, for topping
(optional)

Sliced avocado, for
topping (optional)

Per serving: Calories: 262;
Total fat: 15g; Saturated fat:
3g; Cholesterol: 0mg; Sodium:
377mg; Carbohydrates: 14g;
Fiber: 6g; Sugar: 4g;
Protein: 20g

1. In a large skillet, heat the oil over medium heat. Add the mixed vegetables and garlic and season with a pinch of salt and pepper. Sauté for 5 to 10 minutes, or until the vegetables have softened.

2. Push the vegetables to the sides and use your fingers to crumble the tofu into the center of the pan. Add the salt, turmeric, pepper, and nutritional yeast (if using). Using a spatula, toss the tofu to coat it in the spices. Cook for 5 minutes, or until the tofu is heated through.

3. Add the leafy greens and cook for 2 to 3 minutes, or until they have wilted. If needed, add 2 to 3 teaspoons of water to help them steam. Toss everything to combine.

4. Remove the skillet from the heat and adjust the seasonings as needed. Divide the tofu scramble among four plates and top with hot sauce and avocado slices (if using).

INGREDIENT TIP: If you have extra time in the morning, press your tofu. To do this, wrap the drained block of tofu in paper towels. Place the wrapped block on a plate and place a heavy object on top of the tofu to press it down for at least 15 minutes.

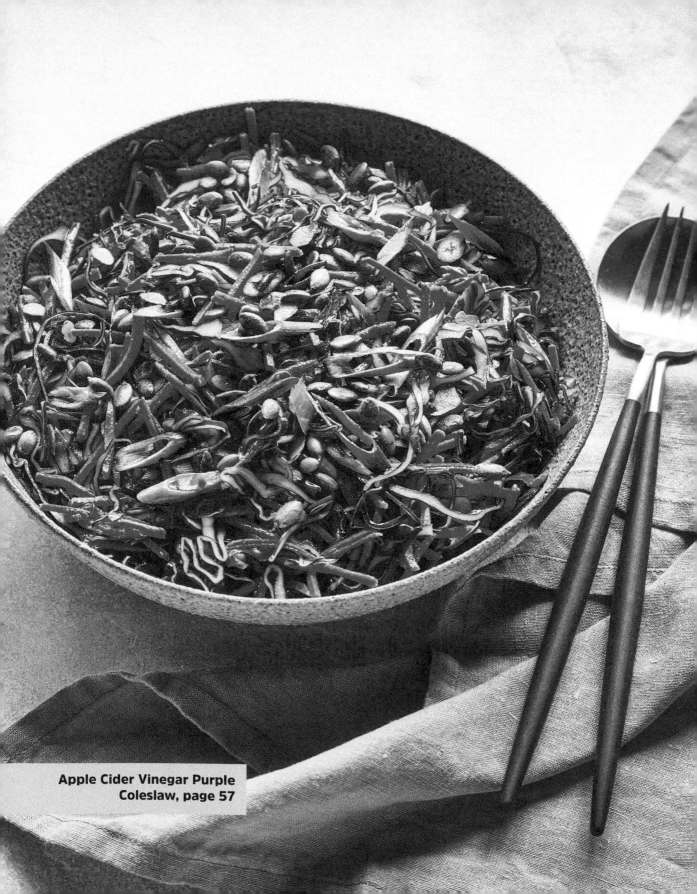

Apple Cider Vinegar Purple
Coleslaw, page 57

CHAPTER 4

Salads, Soups, and Sides

Strawberry and Avocado Salad

SERVES 4 to 6 **PREP TIME**: 10 minutes

30 MINUTES OR LESS | DAIRY-FREE | GLUTEN-FREE | NO-COOK | VEGAN

Basil is a slightly sweet, aromatic herb that's often used to add flavor and color to pizza, pasta, and pesto. It can also add a great depth of flavor to salads. This Strawberry and Avocado Salad will quickly become a summer staple, as it pairs well with a variety of dishes. To turn it into an entrée, add a protein on top, such as grilled tofu or shrimp.

10 ounces fresh baby spinach

½ cup chopped fresh basil

1 pound strawberries, quartered

1 large avocado, diced

½ cup roasted sunflower seeds

½ cup Lemon-Dijon Dressing (page 138)

Per serving: Calories: 265; Total fat: 24g; Saturated fat: 2g; Cholesterol: 0mg; Sodium: 204mg; Carbohydrates: 13g; Fiber: 5g; Sugar: 4g; Protein: 5g

In a large serving bowl, toss together the spinach, basil, strawberries, avocado, and sunflower seeds. Drizzle the dressing over the top just before serving.

SWAP IT: For a small flavor twist, swap out the basil for fresh mint and use a mix of blueberries and raspberries instead of strawberries.

Spring Salmon Salad

SERVES 2 to 4 **PREP TIME**: 10 minutes

5-INGREDIENT | 30 MINUTES OR LESS | DAIRY-FREE | GLUTEN-FREE | NO-COOK

This Spring Salmon Salad is one of my go-tos when I want a nourishing meal that isn't fussy or time-consuming. Despite having just five ingredients, this salad has a lovely variety of flavors and textures and is filled with healthy fats. Although it certainly fits the bill for a light lunch or dinner, I love serving it as part of a weekend brunch with fresh berries and a whole-grain baguette on the side.

5 ounces arugula

3 small Cherry Belle radishes, thinly sliced

6 ounces smoked salmon, sliced

1 small avocado, sliced

¼ cup Lemon-Dijon Dressing (page 138)

Per serving: Calories: 177; Total fat: 14g; Saturated fat: 2g; Cholesterol: 10mg; Sodium: 380mg; Carbohydrates: 5g; Fiber: 3g; Sugar: 1g; Protein: 9g

1. In a large serving bowl, add the arugula. Top with the radishes, salmon, and avocado.

2. Just before serving, drizzle with the dressing.

SWAP IT: Cherry Belle radishes are small, mild cherry-red radishes that are typically in season during the spring and summer. If you're making this salad in the fall or winter, look for watermelon radishes instead.

Massaged Kale Salad

SERVES 4 **PREP TIME**: 20 minutes

30 MINUTES OR LESS | DAIRY-FREE | GLUTEN-FREE | NO-COOK | VEGAN

Kale is often called a superfood because it's incredibly rich in antioxidants, vitamins, and minerals. However, depending on how it's prepared, it can taste bitter. To help reduce the bitterness, there are two key steps you should not skip: Massage the kale and let the salad sit for 10 minutes before eating. Yes, it takes a little bit longer, but I promise the results are worth it!

6 cups chopped Tuscan kale

1 teaspoon freshly squeezed lemon juice

½ teaspoon extra-virgin olive oil

Pinch salt

1 medium Honeycrisp apple, cored and sliced thin

¼ cup chopped pecans, toasted

¼ cup dried cranberries

½ cup Five-Ingredient Ginger Dressing (page 139)

Per serving: Calories: 300; Total fat: 24g; Saturated fat: 3g; Cholesterol: 0mg; Sodium: 249mg; Carbohydrates: 21g; Fiber: 4g; Sugar: 14g; Protein: 4g

1. In a large serving bowl, add the chopped kale and drizzle with the lemon juice, olive oil, and salt. Using your hands, massage the seasoning into the kale leaves for 2 to 3 minutes, or until the leaves become soft and turn a slightly darker shade of green.

2. Add the apple slices, pecans, dried cranberries, and dressing on top. Toss well to combine. For the best flavor, let the salad rest for 10 minutes before serving.

SWAP IT: This salad is best with crisp, slightly tart apples. If you can't find Honeycrisp, other good options include Granny Smith, Pink Lady, and Fuji.

Apple Cider Vinegar Purple Coleslaw

SERVES 6 **PREP TIME**: 15 minutes

30 MINUTES OR LESS | DAIRY-FREE | GLUTEN-FREE | NO-COOK | VEGAN

Coleslaw is a summer staple that's perfect for picnics and barbecues. But because it is often made with mayonnaise, coleslaw isn't always the healthiest choice. This purple coleslaw is a healthier twist, as it subs out the mayo for a tangy vinegar dressing. Enjoy this vibrant recipe as a side dish at your next barbecue or as a topping for Grilled Fish Tacos with Avocado Crema (page 98). This coleslaw can be kept in the refrigerator for up to 5 days.

4 cups shredded purple cabbage

2 cups shredded carrots

¼ cup sliced scallions, green part only

2 tablespoons apple cider vinegar

1 tablespoon pure maple syrup

1 teaspoon Dijon mustard

½ teaspoon salt

¼ teaspoon black pepper

3 tablespoons extra-virgin olive oil

¼ cup roasted pumpkin or sunflower seeds, for garnish (optional)

Per serving: Calories: 139; Total fat: 9g; Saturated fat: 1g; Cholesterol: 0mg; Sodium: 270mg; Carbohydrates: 13g; Fiber: 3g; Sugar: 7g; Protein: 3g

1. In a large serving bowl, combine the cabbage, carrots, and scallions. Set aside.

2. In a small bowl, whisk together the vinegar, maple syrup, mustard, salt, and pepper until well combined. While continuously whisking, slowly pour in the olive oil until it's fully incorporated.

3. Pour the dressing over the slaw and toss well to combine. Taste and adjust the seasonings. Sprinkle the seeds on top (if using).

SWAP IT: Give this coleslaw a Southwestern flair by leaving out the scallions and adding diced jalapeño peppers, chopped fresh cilantro, and a pinch of ground cumin.

Zesty Mayo-Less Potato Salad

SERVES 6 **PREP TIME**: 15 minutes / **COOK TIME**: 5 minutes

30 MINUTES OR LESS | DAIRY-FREE | GLUTEN-FREE | VEGAN

Potato salad is another classic summer recipe that's often loaded with unhealthy fats in the form of mayonnaise and bacon. This healthier version leaves out these traditionally heavy ingredients and instead uses a tangy mustard dressing and fresh parsley. The result is a lighter side dish that's filled with bright and zesty flavors in every bite.

1½ **pounds red potatoes, cut into ¼-inch slices**

¼ **teaspoon salt, plus more for seasoning**

2 **tablespoons apple cider vinegar, divided**

1 **large shallot, diced**

2½ **tablespoons Dijon mustard**

1 **garlic clove, minced**

¼ **teaspoon freshly ground black pepper**

2 **tablespoons red wine vinegar**

3 **tablespoons extra-virgin olive oil**

½ **cup chopped fresh parsley**

Per serving: Calories: 139; Total fat: 9g; Saturated fat: 1g; Cholesterol: 0mg; Sodium: 270mg; Carbohydrates: 13g; Fiber: 3g; Sugar: 7g; Protein: 3g

1. In a large saucepan, combine the potatoes and a pinch of salt. Add enough water to cover the potatoes by 1 inch. Bring them to a boil over high heat, then reduce the heat to medium-low. Cook for 5 minutes, or until the potatoes are easily pierced with a fork. Drain them and place them in a large serving bowl. Toss with 1 tablespoon of apple cider vinegar and the diced shallot. Set aside.

2. In a small bowl, whisk together the mustard, garlic, salt, black pepper, red wine vinegar, and the remaining 1 tablespoon of apple cider vinegar. Whisking continuously, slowly pour in the olive oil until it's fully combined.

3. Pour the dressing over the potatoes and add the parsley. Toss to combine and season with additional salt as desired. Serve warm or refrigerate for at least 1 hour to serve it chilled.

SWAP IT: If you don't have red wine vinegar on hand, you can just use more apple cider vinegar in the recipe instead. Just keep in mind that the flavor won't be quite as complex.

Smashed Avocado and Chickpea Salad

SERVES 4 **PREP TIME**: 10 minutes

5-INGREDIENT | 30 MINUTES OR LESS | DAIRY-FREE | GLUTEN-FREE
NO-COOK | VEGAN

This salad is the ultimate easy yet healthy lunch because it's filled with good fats, protein, and fiber. You'll love this creamy plant-based dish. I recommend serving it as an open-face sandwich on a slice of whole-grain or sourdough bread. You can also spoon it on top of whole-grain crackers, use it as a dip for raw vegetables, or spoon it over a bed of mixed greens.

1 (15-ounce) can chickpeas, drained and rinsed

1 large avocado

2 teaspoons freshly squeezed lemon juice

½ teaspoon paprika

Pinch salt

Pinch freshly ground black pepper

Per serving: Calories: 165; Total fat: 6g; Saturated fat: 1g; Cholesterol: 0mg; Sodium: 66mg; Carbohydrates: 21g; Fiber: 7g; Sugar: 1g; Protein: 6g

1. In a medium bowl, combine the chickpeas, avocado, lemon juice, paprika, salt, and pepper.

2. Using a fork or potato masher, mash the chickpeas and avocado until the mixture is well combined, leaving a few whole chickpeas throughout.

SWAP IT: If you prefer a creamier salad, use white beans instead of the chickpeas.

Quinoa Crunch Salad with Peanut Dressing

SERVES 4 to 6 **PREP TIME**: 10 minutes / **COOK TIME**: 20 minutes

30 MINUTES OR LESS | DAIRY-FREE | GLUTEN-FREE | VEGAN

This quinoa salad is filled with crunchy fresh vegetables and tossed in my Family-Favorite Peanut Sauce for a flavorful side dish that can be made a day ahead of time. (Leftovers will keep in an airtight container in the refrigerator for up to 5 days.) Quinoa is a great source of plant-based protein, so you can also enjoy this grain salad as a side dish or vegan main dish. For even more protein and fiber, add 1 cup of shelled edamame or cooked chickpeas.

¾ cup uncooked quinoa, rinsed

1½ cups water

1 cup shredded purple cabbage

1 red bell pepper, seeded and diced

1 cup shredded carrots

½ cup chopped fresh cilantro

2 scallions, chopped

½ cup cashew halves

Family-Favorite Peanut Sauce (page 141)

Per serving: Calories: 290; Total fat: 18g; Saturated fat: 3g; Cholesterol: 0mg; Sodium: 110mg; Carbohydrates: 24g; Fiber: 4g; Sugar: 5g; Protein: 11g

1. In a medium pot, combine the quinoa and water. Bring to a boil over medium-high heat. Cover the pot with a tight-fitting lid and reduce the heat to medium-low. Simmer for 15 minutes, or until all the water has been absorbed. Remove the pot from the heat and allow the quinoa to cool for 5 minutes with the lid still on.

2. In a large serving bowl, combine the cooked quinoa, purple cabbage, bell pepper, carrot, cilantro, scallions, and cashews. Pour the peanut sauce over the salad and toss well to combine. Serve warm or place in the refrigerator for at least 2 hours to serve it chilled.

MAKE IT EASIER: If you have a food processor, use the shredding blade to quickly shred your cabbage and carrots. You can also buy pre-shredded vegetables to make the prep time even faster.

Nourishing Green Soup

SERVES 6 **PREP TIME**: 10 minutes / **COOK TIME**: 20 minutes

30 MINUTES OR LESS | DAIRY-FREE | GLUTEN-FREE | VEGAN

This nourishing soup has a deep green color and is packed with brain-healthy foods, including broccoli, spinach, and olive oil. For extra texture and even more MIND superfoods, I recommend garnishing your soup with roasted chickpeas, toasted hazelnuts, or cooked white beans. Leftover soup can be stored in an airtight container for up to 4 days in the refrigerator and up to 1 month in the freezer, so make a double batch.

1 tablespoon extra-virgin olive oil

1 medium shallot, minced

2 garlic cloves, minced

2 teaspoons minced fresh ginger, or more

2 medium yellow potatoes, peeled and chopped

1 teaspoon salt

4 cups low-sodium vegetable broth

2 cups broccoli florets

4 cups fresh baby spinach

1 cup unsweetened almond milk

Per serving: Calories: 95; Total fat: 3g; Saturated fat: 0g; Cholesterol: 0mg; Sodium: 536mg; Carbohydrates: 15g; Fiber: 2g; Sugar: 3g; Protein: 3g

1. In a large pot, heat the oil over medium heat. Add the shallot and cook for 2 minutes, or until softened. Add the garlic and ginger. Cook for 1 minute, or until fragrant.

2. Increase the heat to medium-high and stir in the potatoes, salt, and broth. Bring to a boil. Add the broccoli and reduce the heat to medium-low. Simmer for 5 to 7 minutes, or until the broccoli and potatoes are soft. Stir in the spinach and cook for 2 to 3 minutes, or until wilted. Turn off the heat and let the soup cool for 5 minutes.

3. Carefully ladle the soup into a blender (or use an immersion blender) and blend on high until smooth. Pour the blended soup back into the pot and stir in the almond milk. Serve immediately.

SWAP IT: This soup is easily customizable based on what's in season or on sale. Instead of the broccoli, you can use zucchini or asparagus. You can also use another leafy green in place of the spinach, such as kale or Swiss chard.

Curried Carrot Soup

SERVES 2 to 4 **PREP TIME**: 10 minutes / **COOK TIME**: 20 minutes

30 MINUTES OR LESS | DAIRY-FREE | GLUTEN-FREE | VEGAN

Curry powder adds a wonderful warmth and complexity to even the simplest of recipes. I especially love it in this soup, as the slight heat of the curry nicely balances out the sweetness of the carrots. This soup is perfect as a first course or enjoyed on its own with a crusty slice of whole-grain bread on the side. Leftovers will keep for up to 5 days in the refrigerator and up to 4 months in the freezer.

1 tablespoon extra-virgin olive oil

1 large shallot, diced

5 large carrots, peeled and diced

½ cup dried red lentils, rinsed and sorted

2 teaspoons yellow curry powder

1 teaspoon minced fresh ginger, or ½ teaspoon dried ginger

3 cups low-sodium vegetable broth

¼ teaspoon salt

½ cup coconut milk

Per serving: Calories: 185; Total fat: 5g; Saturated fat: 1g; Cholesterol: 0mg; Sodium: 316mg; Carbohydrates: 30g; Fiber: 6g; Sugar: 7g; Protein: 8g

1. In a large pot, heat the oil over medium heat. Add the shallots and carrots. Cook for 5 minutes, or until the carrots begin to soften, stirring frequently.

2. Add the lentils, curry powder, and ginger. Stir to combine and cook for 1 to 2 minutes, or until fragrant. Stir in the vegetable broth and salt. Increase the heat to medium-high and bring the mixture to a boil. Cover the pot with a tight-fitting lid and reduce the heat to medium-low. Simmer for 10 minutes, or until the lentils are soft.

3. Remove the pot from the heat and let the soup cool for 5 minutes. Carefully ladle the soup into a blender and blend on high until smooth.

4. Place the pot back onto the stove over medium heat. Pour the blended soup into the pot and stir in the coconut milk. Cook for another 2 to 3 minutes and adjust the seasonings as desired. Serve immediately.

MAKE IT EASIER: To make pureeing this soup even easier, use an immersion blender. Instead of waiting for the soup to cool and ladling it into a blender, you can puree your soup right in the pot.

Simple Miso Soup

SERVES 4 **PREP TIME**: 5 minutes / **COOK TIME**: 10 minutes

5-INGREDIENT | 30 MINUTES OR LESS | DAIRY-FREE | GLUTEN-FREE | VEGAN

Miso soup is one of my favorite recipes when the weather starts to turn cold because it warms you from the inside out. Traditionally it's made with nori, which are sheets of dried seaweed. However, this recipe uses green chard, which is easier to find and doesn't get as soggy as spinach. If you want the traditional seaweed flavor, add 1 sheet of nori, cut into small rectangles. You can store leftover soup in an airtight container for up to 5 days in the refrigerator or for up to 4 months in the freezer.

4 cups vegetable broth

3 tablespoons white miso paste

½ cup chopped green chard

¼ cup chopped scallions

½ block (7 ounces) firm tofu, pressed, drained, and cubed

Per serving: Calories: 71; Total fat: 2g; Saturated fat: 1g; Cholesterol: 0mg; Sodium: 1203mg; Carbohydrates: 6g; Fiber: 1g; Sugar: 2g; Protein: 7g

1. In a medium pot, bring the vegetable broth to a low simmer over medium heat.

2. In a small bowl, whisk together the miso paste with a spoonful of the hot vegetable broth and set aside.

3. Add the green chard, scallions, and tofu cubes to the pot and cook for 5 minutes, or until the green chard has wilted and the tofu is heated through. Remove from the heat.

4. Whisk the miso into the soup and serve.

SWAP IT: To reduce the sodium in this soup, use low-sodium vegetable broth and season with a pinch of salt. You can also add shiitake mushrooms for extra texture.

Lemon Chicken and Farro Soup

SERVES 4 **PREP TIME**: 10 minutes / **COOK TIME**: 30 minutes

DAIRY-FREE | ONE-POT

This is one of my favorite soups to make, especially as the weather begins to warm up. Although it still has all the comfort of a traditional chicken soup, the addition of fresh lemon juice and zest adds a bright pop of flavor. It also features farro, which is a whole grain with a wonderful chewy texture and a nutty flavor. To make this soup even easier, use a precooked rotisserie chicken to cut down on the prep work.

1 tablespoon extra-virgin olive oil

1 garlic clove, minced

2 large carrots, peeled and chopped

¼ teaspoon freshly ground black pepper

1 teaspoon dried thyme

Zest of ½ small lemon

Juice of 1 small lemon

6 cups low-sodium chicken broth

3 cups cooked chicken breast, cubed

½ cup uncooked pearled farro

Salt

2 cups roughly chopped curly kale

Per serving: Calories: 514; Total fat: 15g; Saturated fat: 4g; Cholesterol: 157mg; Sodium: 320mg; Carbohydrates: 28g; Fiber: 5g; Sugar: 3g; Protein: 68g

1. In a large soup pot, heat the oil over medium-high heat until it's hot and shimmering. Add the garlic and sauté for about 30 seconds, or until fragrant. Then add the carrots, black pepper, thyme, and lemon zest. Cook for 1 minute.

2. Add the lemon juice and chicken broth and increase the heat to high. Bring to a boil. Then reduce the heat to a simmer and add the cooked chicken. Simmer uncovered for 5 minutes, or until the carrots are just starting to soften.

3. Add the farro to the soup and simmer for 15 minutes, or until the farro is soft but still chewy. Taste and season with salt.

4. Finally, add the kale and simmer for 1 to 2 minutes, or until the kale is softened.

MAKE IT EASIER: This recipe calls for pearled farro, which cooks in 15 minutes. Some stores sell farro that cooks in just 10 minutes, which will make this soup even quicker.

Slow-Cooker Turkey and Kale Minestrone Soup

SERVES 6 **PREP TIME**: 10 minutes / **COOK TIME**: 4 hours

DAIRY-FREE | ONE-POT

Minestrone is a hearty Italian soup made with a simple tomato and bean broth. Feel free to use any vegetables you have left over in your refrigerator. This is best served with a crusty slice of bread and a glass of red wine.

1 pound 93-percent lean ground turkey

1 small yellow onion, chopped

2 large carrots, peeled and chopped

1 large celery stalk, chopped

6 cups low-sodium chicken broth

2 (14.5-ounce) cans fire-roasted diced tomatoes, not drained

1 (15-ounce) can no-added-salt white beans, drained and rinsed

½ teaspoon salt

½ teaspoon freshly ground black pepper

1 cup uncooked whole-wheat elbow pasta

2 cups chopped Tuscan or curly kale

1. In a 5- or 6-quart slow cooker, add the turkey. Using a spatula, break up the turkey into crumbles. Stir in the onion, carrots, celery, chicken broth, tomatoes, white beans, salt, and pepper. Cover and cook on low for 3 hours.

2. Stir in the elbow pasta and kale. Continue cooking on low for 1 hour, or until the pasta is soft. Taste and adjust the seasonings before serving.

SWAP IT: To make this soup vegan, leave out the ground turkey and add 2 cups of chopped mixed vegetables, such as zucchini, potatoes, butternut squash, mushrooms, and green beans.

Per serving: Calories: 364; Total fat: 11g; Saturated fat: 3g; Cholesterol: 79mg; Sodium: 986mg; Carbohydrates: 36g; Fiber: 8g; Sugar: 6g; Protein: 35g

Simple Balsamic Roasted Tomatoes

SERVES 4 **PREP TIME**: 10 minutes / **COOK TIME**: 20 minutes

5-INGREDIENT | 30 MINUTES OR LESS | DAIRY-FREE | GLUTEN-FREE | VEGAN

Despite being low in calories, tomatoes are packed with important nutrients, including vitamin C, potassium, and folate. They're also one of the best sources of lycopene, a plant-based compound with antioxidant and anti-inflammatory properties. These Simple Balsamic Roasted Tomatoes are a wonderfully juicy way to enjoy this nutrient-packed fruit. To add a little extra sweetness, add ½ teaspoon of sugar to the tomatoes before roasting. Roasted tomatoes are best the day you make them. However, leftovers can be stored in an airtight container and refrigerated for up to 3 days.

2 pounds cherry tomatoes, cut in half

1½ tablespoons balsamic vinegar

1½ tablespoons extra-virgin olive oil

1 garlic clove, minced

Pinch salt

Per serving: Calories: 102; Total fat: 6g; Saturated fat: 1g; Cholesterol: 0mg; Sodium: 52mg; Carbohydrates: 12g; Fiber: 3g; Sugar: 9g; Protein: 3g

1. Preheat the oven to 350°F. Line a large baking sheet with parchment paper.

2. Place the tomatoes in a large bowl and toss with the balsamic vinegar, olive oil, garlic, and salt.

3. Place the tomatoes on the prepared baking sheet, cut-side down. Roast for 10 minutes. Then rotate the baking sheet and roast for another 10 minutes, or until the tomatoes are soft and releasing their juices. Remove the pan from the oven and let the tomatoes cool for 5 minutes before eating.

SWAP IT: If you can't find cherry tomatoes, you can use grape tomatoes instead, but they won't be quite as juicy.

Go-To Sautéed Garlic Kale

SERVES 4 **PREP TIME**: 10 minutes / **COOK TIME**: 5 minutes

5-INGREDIENT | 30 MINUTES OR LESS | DAIRY-FREE | GLUTEN-FREE
ONE-PAN | VEGAN

If you think you don't like kale, this recipe might just change your mind. Tuscan kale, also called lacinato or dinosaur kale, has dark green, flat leaves. Unlike curly kale, the Tuscan variety has a milder and sweeter flavor. I especially like it roasted, as it reduces the bitterness even more.

2 tablespoons extra-virgin olive oil

2 garlic cloves, smashed

1 pound (2 bunches) Tuscan kale, rinsed, stemmed, and roughly chopped

¼ teaspoon salt

Freshly ground black pepper

Per serving: Calories: 102; Total fat: 8g; Saturated fat: 1g; Cholesterol: 0mg; Sodium: 208mg; Carbohydrates: 6g; Fiber: 5g; Sugar: 1g; Protein: 3g

1. In a large skillet, heat the oil over medium-high heat. Add the garlic and kale. Cook for 3 to 4 minutes, stirring frequently, until the kale is slightly wilted and is a brighter shade of green. Remove from the heat.

2. Stir in the salt and season with pepper. Discard the garlic cloves and serve hot.

INGREDIENT TIP: If you're cooking for picky eaters or still find the kale to be a bit too bitter, drizzle some fresh lemon juice on top just before serving.

The Best Roasted Vegetables

SERVES 6 **PREP TIME**: 15 minutes / **COOK TIME**: 35 minutes

DAIRY-FREE | GLUTEN-FREE | ONE-PAN | VEGAN

Every home cook should have a go-to roasted vegetable recipe. This particular recipe is a staple in my house because the seasonings aren't too overpowering, making it a perfectly versatile side dish. However, when I'm feeling a little more decadent, I like to add a drizzle of balsamic glaze over the vegetables after roasting. Store leftover roasted vegetables in an airtight container for up to 5 days in the refrigerator.

2 large carrots, peeled and cut into 1-inch chunks

½ pound Brussels sprouts, outer leaves removed, sliced in half

1 pound sweet potatoes, peeled and cut into 1-inch-thick slices

¼ cup extra-virgin olive oil

2 teaspoons dried oregano

2 teaspoons dried rosemary

1 teaspoon dried basil

½ teaspoon salt

½ teaspoon freshly ground black pepper

Per serving: Calories: 174; Total fat: 9g; Saturated fat: 1g; Cholesterol: 0mg; Sodium: 265mg; Carbohydrates: 22g; Fiber: 5g; Sugar: 5g; Protein: 3g

1. Preheat the oven to 400°F. Line a large baking sheet with parchment paper.

2. Place the carrots, Brussels sprouts, and sweet potatoes on the prepared baking sheet in an even layer. If you can't fit all the vegetables without overlapping, either use a second pan or roast the vegetables in batches. Drizzle with the olive oil and sprinkle with the oregano, rosemary, basil, salt, and pepper. Toss to coat.

3. Roast the vegetables for 35 minutes, tossing halfway through. Remove the pan from the oven and allow the vegetables to cool slightly before serving.

SWAP IT: Use any vegetables that are in season or already in your refrigerator. Onions, baby potatoes, butternut squash cubes, asparagus, portobello mushrooms, cauliflower, and broccoli all work particularly well.

Lemony Brown Rice

SERVES 6 **PREP TIME**: 5 minutes / **COOK TIME**: 40 minutes

5-INGREDIENT | DAIRY-FREE | GLUTEN-FREE | ONE-POT | VEGAN

When you need a simple side dish, look no further than this recipe. Lightly flavored with fresh parsley and lemon juice, this fluffy rice goes perfectly alongside almost any entrée. I recommend pairing it with the Fish en Papillote with Summer Squash (page 99) or the Strawberry-Balsamic Chicken (page 112). If you're short on time, use a quick-cooking brown rice.

1 cup uncooked brown rice, rinsed

1¾ cups low-sodium vegetable broth

1 tablespoon extra-virgin olive oil

Zest and juice of 1 medium lemon

2 tablespoons finely chopped fresh parsley

Per serving: Calories: 139; Total fat: 3g; Saturated fat: 1g; Cholesterol: 0mg; Sodium: 42mg; Carbohydrates: 25g; Fiber: 1g; Sugar: 1g; Protein: 3g

1. In a medium pot over high heat, combine the brown rice, vegetable broth, and olive oil. Bring to a boil. Cover the pot with a tight-fitting lid and reduce the heat to medium-low. Simmer for 35 minutes, or until the rice is soft.

2. Remove the pot from the heat. Fluff the rice with a fork and stir in the lemon zest, lemon juice, and parsley. Serve warm.

SWAP IT: Replace the parsley with other herbs depending on what you'll be serving the rice with. For example, use dill for Greek-inspired or fish recipes, cilantro for Mexican-inspired recipes, or mint for Thai- or Indian-inspired dishes.

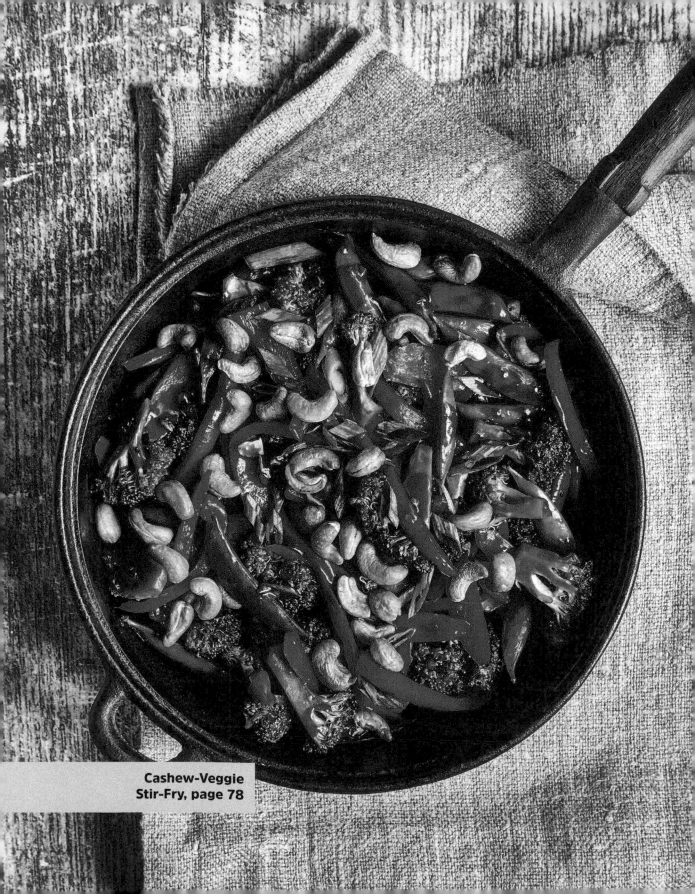

Cashew-Veggie
Stir-Fry, page 78

CHAPTER 5

Vegan and Vegetarian Mains

Lemon Grain Bowls with Cracked Freekeh and Roasted Chickpeas

SERVES 4 **PREP TIME**: 10 minutes / **COOK TIME**: 20 minutes

30 MINUTES OR LESS | DAIRY-FREE | VEGAN

Freekeh is a Middle Eastern whole grain that's made from toasted wheat. When cooked, it has a delicious nutty, slightly buttery flavor that goes well in dishes that aren't heavily spiced. I particularly love using it in vegetarian and vegan recipes because freekeh is high in fiber and protein. Just make sure to buy cracked freekeh because it cooks faster.

2 medium zucchini, thinly sliced

½ pint cherry tomatoes, halved

1 (15-ounce) can chickpeas, drained and rinsed

2 tablespoons extra-virgin olive oil

Salt

Freshly ground black pepper

1 cup cracked freekeh

2½ cups low-sodium vegetable broth

Juice of 1 medium lemon

Per serving: Calories: 387; Total fat: 12g; Saturated fat: 1g; Cholesterol: 0mg; Sodium: 393mg; Carbohydrates: 62g; Fiber: 13g; Sugar: 11g; Protein: 16g

1. Preheat the oven to 350°F. Line a large baking sheet with parchment paper.

2. In a large bowl, combine the zucchini, tomatoes, and chickpeas. Toss the vegetables with olive oil and season with a pinch of salt and pepper.

3. Spread the mixture out on the prepared baking sheet in an even layer. Roast for 20 minutes, or until the zucchini and tomatoes are lightly browned and the chickpeas are slightly crispy. Remove from the oven.

4. While the zucchini mixture is roasting, in a medium pot over high heat, combine the freekeh and vegetable broth. Bring to a boil, then cover the pot with a tight-fitting lid. Reduce the heat to medium-low and simmer for 15 minutes, or until the freekeh is soft but still chewy. Remove from the heat.

5. In a large serving bowl, stir together the cooked freekeh and the roasted zucchini, tomatoes, and chickpeas. Drizzle the lemon juice on top and stir again to combine. Serve immediately.

SWAP IT: To make this grain bowl gluten-free, use quinoa or buckwheat groats instead of freekeh.

Tofu-Spinach Curry

SERVES 4 **PREP TIME**: 10 minutes / **COOK TIME**: 35 minutes

DAIRY-FREE | GLUTEN-FREE | ONE-POT | VEGAN

This recipe is based on *saag paneer*, a classic Indian curry. Paneer, a type of soft Indian cheese, is delicious but not terribly MIND diet–friendly. Instead, I use protein-rich tofu for a similar texture and an equally tasty and satisfying dish. Serve with brown rice or whole-wheat flatbread.

3 tablespoons extra-virgin olive oil, divided

1 (14-ounce) package firm tofu, drained and cubed

2 plum tomatoes, chopped

1 teaspoon minced fresh ginger

¼ teaspoon ground cumin

½ teaspoon ground turmeric

¼ teaspoon cayenne pepper

10 ounces frozen spinach, thawed and squeezed to remove excess liquid

½ teaspoon salt

1½ cups light coconut milk

Per serving: Calories: 275; Total fat: 23g; Saturated fat: 10g; Cholesterol: 0mg; Sodium: 383mg; Carbohydrates: 9g; Fiber: 5g; Sugar: 3g; Protein: 11g

1. In a large skillet, heat the oil over medium-high heat. When the oil is hot, add the tofu and cook for 10 minutes, flipping the cubes occasionally. You want all four sides of each cube to get lightly browned. Remove from the pan and set aside.

2. In a blender, blend the tomatoes and ginger until they form a smooth puree. Pour the tomato mixture into the skillet and set the heat to medium. Stir in the cumin, turmeric, and cayenne pepper. Cook for 5 to 7 minutes, or until the mixture is reduced by nearly half.

3. Add the spinach and salt and cook for 10 minutes. Stir in the coconut milk and seared tofu. Cook for another 5 minutes, or until the tofu is heated through.

MAKE IT EASIER: To save time and enhance the flavor of this dish, make the spinach curry the night before and then reheat it while you brown the tofu.

One-Pan Southwestern Quinoa Skillet

SERVES 4 **PREP TIME**: 10 minutes / **COOK TIME**: 25 minutes

DAIRY-FREE | GLUTEN-FREE | ONE-PAN | VEGAN

This one-pan dish is an easy weeknight meal for the whole family. Made with Southwestern spices, including chili powder and cumin, it gets even better when topped with fresh avocado, salsa, and a squeeze of lime juice. You can enjoy this recipe as a grain bowl or use it as a filling for easy, plant-based burritos. It will keep in the refrigerator in an airtight container for up to 5 days.

1 tablespoon extra-virgin olive oil

2 garlic cloves, minced

1 medium jalapeño pepper, seeded and diced

1½ teaspoons chili powder

½ teaspoon ground cumin

1 large zucchini, diced

1 large bell pepper, seeded and diced

1 pint cherry tomatoes, halved

1 (15-ounce) can no-added-salt black beans, drained and rinsed

1 cup uncooked quinoa, rinsed

1¼ cups vegetable broth

Salt

Freshly ground black pepper

1. In a large skillet, heat the oil over medium heat until it is hot and shimmering. Add the garlic and jalapeño and sauté for 30 seconds, stirring frequently.

2. Add the chili powder, cumin, zucchini, bell pepper, tomatoes, and black beans. Stir well to combine. Next, add the quinoa and broth. Stir the mixture, making sure to scrape the bottom of the pan in case any vegetables or beans are sticking to the bottom.

3. Increase the heat to high and bring to a boil, then reduce the heat to low and cover. Simmer for 20 minutes, or until the quinoa is soft and fluffy. Season with salt and pepper.

Avocado slices, for serving (optional)

Salsa, for serving (optional)

Fresh lime wedges, for serving (optional)

Per serving: Calories: 302; Total fat: 8g; Saturated fat: 1g; Cholesterol: 0mg; Sodium: 294mg; Carbohydrates: 50g; Fiber: 10g; Sugar: 12g; Protein: 11g

4. Serve with avocado slices, salsa, and fresh lime wedges.

SWAP IT: Use any combination of vegetables that are in season or that you have left over in the refrigerator. Broccoli and cauliflower, for example, would work nicely.

Quinoa-Stuffed Sweet Potatoes

SERVES 4 **PREP TIME**: 10 minutes / **COOK TIME**: 20 minutes

30 MINUTES OR LESS | DAIRY-FREE | GLUTEN-FREE | VEGAN

While we often pair them with sweeter toppings, like cinnamon or brown sugar, sweet potatoes also provide a nice contrast to more savory Mediterranean flavors. Cook a large batch of sweet potatoes over the weekend to eat throughout the week as a side or for breakfast. Toward the end of the week, whip up this quinoa filling and reheat a potato for a quick weeknight dinner.

⅔ cup uncooked quinoa, rinsed

1⅓ cups low-sodium vegetable broth

4 medium sweet potatoes

2 tablespoons extra-virgin olive oil

4 cups fresh baby spinach

Salt

Black pepper

1 (15-ounce) can chickpeas, drained and rinsed

½ cup sun-dried tomatoes, chopped

½ teaspoon dried thyme

½ teaspoon garlic powder

Simple Tzatziki (page 142, optional)

Per serving: Calories: 453; Total fat: 12g; Saturated fat: 2g; Cholesterol: 0mg; Sodium: 450mg; Carbohydrates: 74g; Fiber: 14g; Sugar: 15g; Protein: 16g

1. In a medium pot over high heat, combine the quinoa and broth. Bring to a boil. Cover the pot with a tight-fitting lid and reduce the heat to medium-low. Simmer for 15 minutes, or until the broth has been absorbed. Set aside.

2. Meanwhile, poke a few holes in each sweet potato using a fork and place them on a microwave-safe plate. Microwave the sweet potatoes for 10 to 12 minutes, or until soft. Set aside.

3. In a medium skillet, heat the oil over medium heat. Add the spinach and season with a pinch of salt and pepper. Cook for 2 to 3 minutes, or until the spinach has wilted. Stir in the cooked quinoa, chickpeas, sun-dried tomatoes, thyme, and garlic powder. Taste and add more salt or pepper as needed. Remove from the heat and set aside.

4. Cut each sweet potato in half and top with the quinoa mixture. Drizzle tzatziki sauce over top (if using).

MAKE IT EASIER: Instead of tzatziki, mix plain Greek yogurt (or a plant-based yogurt alternative) with fresh or dried dill and a splash of lemon juice for a quick and easy topping.

Salsa Verde Enchiladas

SERVES 4 **PREP TIME**: 10 minutes / **COOK TIME**: 20 minutes

5-INGREDIENT | 30 MINUTES OR LESS | DAIRY-FREE | GLUTEN-FREE | VEGAN

While enchiladas traditionally are smothered in cheese, this recipe is a healthier plant-based version. All you need are five ingredients and half an hour for a simple yet flavor-packed meal. Feel free to add your own twist with a variety of toppings, such as guacamole, plant-based sour cream, or sliced jalapeño peppers. You can make them even heartier by adding left-over roasted vegetables to the filling. Store leftovers in an airtight container for up to 5 days in the refrigerator.

1 (16-ounce) package extra-firm tofu, drained and pressed, cut into cubes

1 (15-ounce) can no-added-salt black beans, drained and rinsed

2 tablespoons low-sodium taco seasoning

2 cups salsa verde, divided

12 small corn tortillas

Per serving: Calories: 403; Total fat: 9g; Saturated fat: 2g; Cholesterol: 0mg; Sodium: 1478mg; Carbohydrates: 61g; Fiber: 11g; Sugar: 7g; Protein: 23g

1. Preheat the oven to 375°F.

2. In a medium bowl, combine the cubed tofu, black beans, taco seasoning, and ½ cup of salsa verde.

3. Divide the tofu mixture evenly among the 12 tortillas. Roll up each tortilla and place it in a 9-by-9-inch baking pan, seam-side down. Pour the remaining 1½ cups of salsa over the top of the enchiladas and bake for 20 minutes.

4. Remove the baked enchiladas from the oven and cool for 5 minutes before serving.

SWAP IT: Salsa verde is made from tomatillos and has a tangy, citrus-like flavor that adds a bright boost of flavor. However, you can use 2 cups of red enchilada sauce instead.

Cashew-Veggie Stir-Fry

SERVES 4 **PREP TIME**: 10 minutes / **COOK TIME**: 20 minutes

30 MINUTES OR LESS | DAIRY-FREE | GLUTEN-FREE | VEGAN

Whether you're new to cooking or just in need of a quick and easy meal, stir-fries are a great option. Not only do they come together quickly, but they're also a great way to use up any leftover vegetables you have in your refrigerator or freezer. For a balanced meal, serve this stir-fry over brown rice or brown rice noodles.

¼ cup low-sodium soy sauce, gluten-free if needed

2 tablespoons maple syrup

2 teaspoons cornstarch

1 tablespoon grated fresh ginger

1 garlic clove, minced

½ cup raw cashews

1 tablespoon extra-virgin olive oil

2 bell peppers, any color, seeded and sliced

1 cup sugar snap peas

2 large carrots, sliced

2 cups broccoli florets

2 scallions, sliced, white and green parts separated (optional)

Per serving: Calories: 213; Total fat: 11g; Saturated fat: 2g; Cholesterol: 0mg; Sodium: 617mg; Carbohydrates: 24g; Fiber: 5g; Sugar: 11g; Protein: 7g

1. To make the sauce, in a small bowl, whisk together the soy sauce, maple syrup, cornstarch, ginger, and garlic. Set aside.

2. In a large wok or skillet, heat the cashews over medium-high heat, stirring frequently. Cook until the cashews are lightly toasted, about 3 to 5 minutes. Remove from the pan and set aside.

3. Add the olive oil to the pan. When the oil is hot, add the bell peppers, snap peas, carrots, broccoli, and the white parts of the scallions (if using). Cook for 8 to 10 minutes, or until the vegetables are slightly soft but still crispy, stirring frequently.

4. Add the stir-fry sauce and cook until the sauce has slightly thickened, about 3 minutes. Remove the skillet from the heat and add the cashews and green parts of the scallions (if using) on top.

SWAP IT: For extra protein, add cubed tofu, shelled edamame, or chickpeas to your stir-fry. For a non-vegan option, you can also add shrimp, salmon, or chicken.

White Bean and Collard Greens Skillet

SERVES 4 **PREP TIME**: 10 minutes / **COOK TIME**: 20 minutes

30 MINUTES OR LESS | DAIRY-FREE | VEGAN

A staple in Southern dishes, collard greens get a unique smoky flavor when cooked. To help balance out the flavors of this dish, we're adding lemon juice and tomatoes for a pop of acidity. For even more flavor, sprinkle red pepper flakes or nutritional yeast over the greens just before serving.

3 cups low-sodium vegetable broth

1 cup uncooked pearled farro

1 tablespoon extra-virgin olive oil

1 large shallot, diced

2 garlic cloves, minced

1 bunch collard greens, stemmed and roughly chopped

Juice of 1 large lemon (about 3 tablespoons)

Salt

Freshly ground black pepper

1 (15-ounce) can no-added-salt cannellini beans, drained and rinsed

1 (14-ounce) can diced tomatoes

Per serving: Calories: 346; Total fat: 5g; Saturated fat: 1g; Cholesterol: 0mg; Sodium: 348mg; Carbohydrates: 65g; Fiber: 14g; Sugar: 6g; Protein: 15g

1. In a medium pot over high heat, add the vegetable broth and bring to a boil. Then stir in the farro and reduce the heat to medium. Simmer for 15 to 20 minutes, or until the farro is soft but chewy. Remove the pot from the heat and set aside.

2. In a large skillet, heat the oil over medium heat. Add the shallot and sauté for 2 to 3 minutes, or until softened. Add the garlic and sauté for 1 minute. Then add the collard greens and lemon juice and season with a pinch of salt and pepper. Cook for 4 minutes, or until the collard greens are starting to soften.

3. Stir in the cannellini beans and tomatoes and season with another pinch of salt and pepper. Cook for 5 minutes, or until the mixture is heated through and the collard greens are starting to wilt.

4. Serve the collard greens over the cooked farro and enjoy immediately.

SWAP IT: Especially during the summer when they're in season, I recommend using 2 fresh Roma or heirloom tomatoes instead of canned for even better flavor.

Spanish Spinach with Chickpeas

SERVES 4 **PREP TIME**: 5 minutes / **COOK TIME**: 10 minutes

30 MINUTES OR LESS | DAIRY-FREE | GLUTEN-FREE | ONE-POT | VEGAN

Chickpeas and spinach is a classic Spanish tapas dish that's made with just a handful of wholesome ingredients. Although it's often served over crusty bread as an appetizer, it can easily be turned into a vegan entrée by serving the sautéed spinach and chickpeas over a bowl of brown rice. Store leftovers in an airtight container in the refrigerator for up to 3 days.

1 tablespoon extra-virgin olive oil

6 garlic cloves, minced

1 teaspoon paprika

½ teaspoon ground cumin

10 ounces fresh baby spinach

2 (15-ounce) cans chickpeas, drained and rinsed

Salt

Freshly ground black pepper

⅓ cup toasted pine nuts, for garnish

Per serving: Calories: 422; Total fat: 17g; Saturated fat: 2g; Cholesterol: 0mg; Sodium: 555mg; Carbohydrates: 55g; Fiber: 17g; Sugar: 10g; Protein: 19g

1. In a large pan, heat the oil over medium-high heat. Stir in the garlic, paprika, and cumin. Cook for 1 minute, or until the spices are fragrant.

2. Reduce the heat to medium and add the spinach. Cook for 3 to 4 minutes, or until the spinach has wilted. Stir in the chickpeas and cook for another 2 to 3 minutes, or until the chickpeas are warmed through. Taste and season with salt and pepper. Remove the skillet from the heat.

3. Garnish with toasted pine nuts and enjoy hot.

SWAP IT: There are many variations of this recipe. Other ingredients you can add include dried raisins, fresh or canned tomatoes, or a splash of white wine. If you can't find pine nuts, roasted hazelnuts or toasted almonds will also work well here.

Mushroom Pasta with Sautéed Spinach

SERVES 6 **PREP TIME**: 10 minutes / **COOK TIME**: 15 minutes

30 MINUTES OR LESS | DAIRY-FREE | VEGAN

Mushrooms are a rich source of essential vitamins and minerals, as well as protective antioxidants. In fact, a 2019 study by Feng et al. published in the *Journal of Alzheimer's Disease* found a link between eating mushrooms twice a week and having a reduced risk of cognitive decline.

6 quarts water

Salt

12 ounces whole-wheat linguini

3 tablespoons extra-virgin olive oil

1 large shallot, diced

2 garlic cloves, minced

3 cups sliced button mushrooms

1 tablespoon low-sodium soy sauce

½ cup low-sodium vegetable broth

10 ounces fresh baby spinach

Freshly ground black pepper

2 teaspoons freshly squeezed lime juice

½ cup chopped fresh parsley, for garnish

¼ cup toasted pine nuts, for garnish (optional)

Per serving: Calories: 235; Total fat: 2g; Saturated fat: 0g; Cholesterol: 0mg; Sodium: 177mg; Carbohydrates: 48g; Fiber: 7g; Sugar: 4g; Protein: 11g

1. In a large pot over high heat, add the water and season with a pinch of salt. Bring to a boil, then carefully add the linguini and cook for 7 minutes, or until al dente. Drain and set the cooked pasta aside.

2. In a large skillet, heat the oil over medium heat. When the oil is hot, add the shallots and garlic. Sauté for 2 to 3 minutes, or until the shallots are softened. Add the mushrooms and cook for 3 minutes, or until lightly browned. Add the soy sauce and vegetable broth. Reduce the heat to medium-low and cook for 2 minutes. Add the spinach and cook for another 2 to 3 minutes, or until it has wilted. Season with a pinch of salt and pepper.

3. Add the cooked pasta to the skillet and toss to combine. Remove the skillet from the heat and add the lime juice. Top with the fresh parsley and toasted pine nuts (if using) and serve immediately.

SWAP IT: While button mushrooms are one of the easiest to find, you can use another variety. I recommend either shiitake mushrooms, as they'll lend a slight smoky flavor, or oyster mushrooms, which are sweeter and more delicate.

Black Bean–Sweet Potato Burgers

SERVES 6 **PREP TIME**: 15 minutes / **COOK TIME**: 10 minutes

30 MINUTES OR LESS | DAIRY-FREE | VEGAN

Forget the dry veggie burgers you've had in the past. These Black Bean–Sweet Potato Burgers are crispy on the outside and soft and moist on the inside. Perfect for kids and adults! You can serve these patties with whole-wheat buns or add them to salads for a lower-carb option. To make these on a grill, it's best to make and form the patties a day ahead of time and let them chill in the refrigerator overnight. This will help them keep their shape when grilling. Lightly oil the patties before grilling and cook for 4 to 5 minutes per side. Store leftover cooked patties in an airtight container for up to 5 days in the refrigerator. Leftovers are best reheated on the stove.

1 medium sweet potato, cooked

1 (15-ounce) can black beans, drained and rinsed

½ cup old-fashioned rolled oats

1 teaspoon ground cumin

1 teaspoon paprika

½ teaspoon garlic powder

1 teaspoon salt

2 tablespoons extra-virgin olive oil

6 whole-wheat burger buns

1. In a large bowl, mash the sweet potato using a fork or potato masher until it's mostly smooth. Add the black beans and continue to mash, leaving a few beans whole. Add the oats, cumin, paprika, garlic powder, and salt and mix well to combine.

2. Using a ½-cup measuring cup, scoop the bean burger mixture and form it into 6 patties, each about ½-inch thick. Place the formed patties on a cutting board and set aside.

3. In a large skillet or griddle, heat the oil over medium-high heat. Carefully add the patties and cook for 4 to 5 minutes, or until the bottoms are lightly browned. Flip and cook for another 4 to 5 minutes, or until lightly browned. Remove from the heat. Depending on the size of your skillet, you may need to cook 3 patties at a time or use two skillets.

Continued ▶

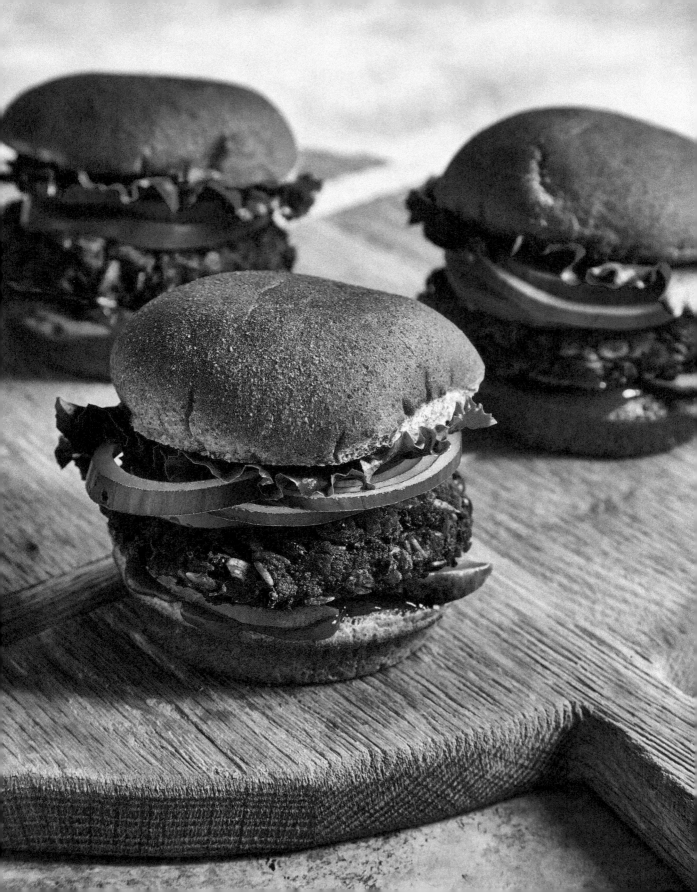

Optional toppings

Lettuce

Tomato slices

Avocado slices

Chopped onions

Ketchup

Barbecue sauce

Per serving: Calories: 426; Total fat: 14g; Saturated fat: 2g; Cholesterol: 0mg; Sodium: 455mg; Carbohydrates: 62g; Fiber: 14g; Sugar: 12g; Protein: 16g

4. Serve immediately on the whole-wheat buns with the toppings of your choice.

SWAP IT: You can use white or pinto beans instead of the black beans. You can also add ¼ cup of sunflower or pumpkin seeds to the patty mixture for added crunch.

Crispy Baked Tofu and Broccoli Noodle Bowls

SERVES 4 **PREP TIME**: 10 minutes / **COOK TIME**: 20 minutes

30 MINUTES OR LESS | DAIRY-FREE | GLUTEN-FREE | VEGAN

This crispy tofu recipe hits all the right notes to be considered a truly comforting dish: crispy and creamy, sweet and salty. Although the peanut sauce comes together quickly, you can also make it a day or two ahead of time and then reheat it on the stove or in the microwave.

1 (14-ounce) package extra-firm tofu, drained and pressed, cut into cubes

4 cups chopped broccoli florets

3 tablespoons extra-virgin olive oil

½ teaspoon garlic powder

¼ teaspoon ground ginger

Salt

Freshly ground black pepper

2 quarts water

8 ounces uncooked brown rice noodles

½ cup Family-Favorite Peanut Sauce (page 141)

Lime wedges, for serving (optional)

Per serving: Calories: 517; Total fat: 25g; Saturated fat: 4g; Cholesterol: 0mg; Sodium: 140mg; Carbohydrates: 53g; Fiber: 6g; Sugar: 2g; Protein: 20g

1. Preheat the oven to 425°F. Line a large baking sheet with parchment paper.

2. In a large bowl, combine the cubed tofu and broccoli. Add the olive oil, garlic powder, and ginger and season with a pinch of salt and pepper. Toss to combine.

3. Spread the tofu and vegetables on the prepared baking sheet in an even layer. Bake for 10 minutes, stir, and bake for another 10 minutes.

4. While the tofu and vegetables are cooking, in a medium pot, bring the water to a boil over high heat. Remove the pot from the heat and stir in the brown rice noodles. Let the noodles soak for 5 minutes, or until they are tender but chewy. Drain and place the cooked noodles in a large bowl. Set aside.

5. Transfer the roasted tofu and broccoli to the bowl with the cooked noodles and add the peanut sauce. Toss to combine. Serve with lime wedges (if using) and enjoy hot.

SWAP IT: For extra vegetables and nutrition, you can use spiralized sweet potatoes or riced cauliflower in place of the brown rice noodles. If you have leftover brown rice or another cooked whole grain, you can use that, as well.

White Bean and Veggie Quinoa Bowls with Pesto

SERVES 4 **PREP TIME**: 10 minutes / **COOK TIME**: 20 minutes

30 MINUTES OR LESS | DAIRY-FREE | GLUTEN-FREE | VEGAN

These quinoa bowls are more of an idea than a strict recipe. Feel free to use any leftover vegetables in your refrigerator and swap the white beans with chickpeas or cooked tofu. Top these grain bowls with Vegan Spinach Pesto (page 144), which can also be made a day ahead of time.

1 small head broccoli, cut into florets

1 medium head cauliflower, cut into florets

5 large carrots, peeled and sliced

3 tablespoons extra-virgin olive oil

1 teaspoon garlic powder

1 teaspoon paprika

½ teaspoon salt

½ teaspoon freshly ground black pepper

1 cup uncooked quinoa, rinsed

2 cups water

1 (15-ounce) can cannellini beans, drained and rinsed

Vegan Spinach Pesto (page 144)

Per serving: Calories: 295; Total fat: 7g; Saturated fat: 1g; Cholesterol: 0mg; Sodium: 875mg; Carbohydrates: 46g; Fiber: 12g; Sugar: 3g; Protein: 13g

1. Preheat the oven to 425°F. Line a large baking sheet with parchment paper.

2. Place the broccoli, cauliflower, and carrots on the prepared baking sheet. Toss the vegetables with the olive oil, garlic powder, paprika, salt, and pepper. Roast for 10 minutes, flip the vegetables, and roast for another 10 minutes. Remove from the oven and set aside.

3. While the vegetables are roasting, in a medium pot over high heat, combine the quinoa and water. Bring to a boil and then cover with a tight-fitting lid. Reduce the heat to medium-low and simmer for 15 minutes, or until all the water has been absorbed. Once cooked, use a fork to fluff the quinoa. Stir in the white beans.

4. To assemble, evenly distribute the roasted vegetables and quinoa among four serving bowls. Top each bowl with 1 to 2 tablespoons of pesto, or more to taste.

MAKE IT EASIER: To save time, you can also use a store-bought pesto. Just note that most premade pesto contains cheese, which is a food that's limited on the MIND diet.

Mediterranean Roasted Veggie Wraps

SERVES 4 **PREP TIME**: 10 minutes / **COOK TIME**: 20 minutes

30 MINUTES OR LESS | DAIRY-FREE | VEGAN

Wraps are the perfect lunch option because they're portable and it's easy to make a big batch of the filling at the beginning of the week. I especially like Mediterranean veggie wraps because you get a variety of textures and flavors without needing a long list of ingredients. Although this recipe calls for roasted zucchini, eggplant would also be delicious and would give this dish a meatier texture. I recommend serving your wrap with a dollop of Simple Tzatziki (page 142) on the side.

2 large zucchini

1 tablespoon extra-virgin olive oil

2 teaspoons paprika

Salt

Freshly ground black pepper

4 whole-wheat tortillas

1 (15-ounce) can cannellini beans, drained and rinsed

1 cup cooked quinoa

1 large Roma tomato, sliced

Per serving: Calories: 356; Total fat: 8g; Saturated fat: 1g; Cholesterol: 0mg; Sodium: 341mg; Carbohydrates: 59g; Fiber: 11g; Sugar: 7g; Protein: 14g

1. Preheat the oven to 375°F. Line a baking sheet with parchment paper.

2. Slice each zucchini lengthwise into 4 slices. Place the zucchini slices on the prepared baking sheet and drizzle the olive oil over top. Sprinkle with the paprika, season with salt and pepper, and toss to evenly coat. Roast the zucchini for 15 to 20 minutes, or until the zucchini is soft and lightly browned. Remove the pan from the oven.

3. To assemble the wraps, place two roasted zucchini slices in the middle of each tortilla. Top with the cannellini beans, cooked quinoa, and tomato slices. Roll each wrap tightly and enjoy immediately.

MAKE IT EASIER: To make this a no-cook wrap, use sliced cucumber instead of the roasted zucchini.

Baked Lentil Meatballs

SERVES 4 **PREP TIME**: 15 minutes, plus 15 minutes to chill / **COOK TIME**: 15 minutes

5-INGREDIENT | DAIRY-FREE | GLUTEN-FREE | VEGETARIAN

Whether you're looking for a meatless alternative to meatballs or want a new way to enjoy lentils, this recipe is a great base for a variety of meals. I like eating these with my Hidden Veggie Marinara Sauce over whole-wheat pasta, but you could also toss these meatless meatballs in Buffalo sauce and use them as a filling for a wrap.

1 cup old-fashioned rolled oats, gluten-free if needed

2 cups cooked or canned green lentils

2 large eggs, lightly beaten

½ teaspoon salt

¼ teaspoon freshly ground black pepper

Hidden Veggie Marinara Sauce (page 145)

Per serving: Calories: 317; Total fat: 8g; Saturated fat: 2g; Cholesterol: 82mg; Sodium: 656mg; Carbohydrates: 47g; Fiber: 12g; Sugar: 9g; Protein: 16g

1. In a food processor, pulse the oats until they reach a coarse bread crumb–like consistency. Transfer them to a large bowl.

2. Add the lentils, eggs, salt, and pepper to the bowl and mix until well combined. Transfer 2 cups of the mixture to the food processor and pulse a few times until nearly smooth. Pour the pulsed mixture back into the bowl and stir to combine. Place the bowl in the freezer for 15 minutes. The mixture should still be soft but firm enough to form a ball.

3. While the lentil meatball mixture is in the freezer, preheat the oven to 375°F. Line a large baking sheet with parchment paper.

4. Using a spoon, scoop up the meatball mixture and roll it into golf ball–size balls. You should get about 20 meatballs. Place the lentil meatballs on the prepared baking sheet and bake for 12 minutes, or until the tops are slightly hardened. Remove from the oven.

5. Toss the lentil meatballs with the marinara sauce and enjoy immediately.

SWAP IT: For Italian-style dishes, add 1 tablespoon of dried Italian seasoning and 1 to 2 tablespoons of chopped fresh herbs, like basil or Italian parsley, to the lentil mixture. You can also use 1 cup of bread crumbs in place of the rolled oats.

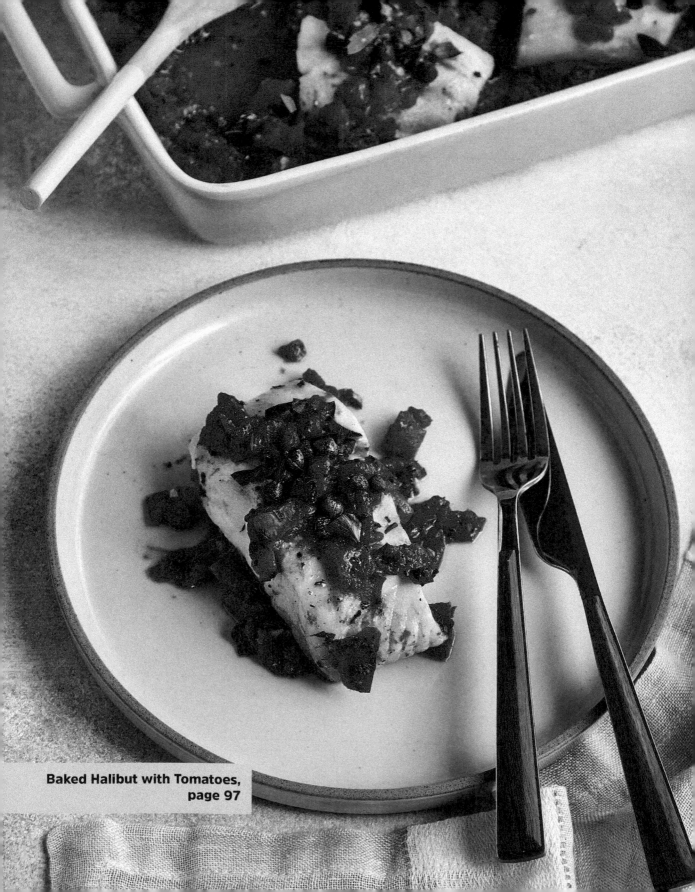

Baked Halibut with Tomatoes, page 97

CHAPTER 6

Fish and Seafood Mains

Mayo-Less Apple Tuna Salad Sandwich

SERVES 4 **PREP TIME**: 10 minutes

5-INGREDIENT | 30 MINUTES OR LESS | GLUTEN-FREE | NO-COOK

Tuna salad is the perfect easy lunch. If you don't want to make a sandwich, you can also spread this on whole-grain crackers or add it on top of mixed greens for a salad. This recipe is a healthier twist, as it uses plain Greek yogurt in place of mayonnaise. It also uses diced apple for a great crunch and touch of sweetness. Crisp, tart apples such as Pink Lady, Honeycrisp, Fuji, or Granny Smith work best. This salad will keep in the refrigerator for up to 4 days.

4 (5-ounce) cans albacore tuna, drained

1 medium apple, cored and diced small

½ cup low-fat plain Greek yogurt

1 tablespoon Dijon mustard

8 slices whole-grain bread

Per serving: Calories: 396; Total fat: 8g; Saturated fat: 1g; Cholesterol: 57mg; Sodium: 466mg; Carbohydrates: 42g; Fiber: 7g; Sugar: 10g; Protein: 44g

1. In a large bowl, combine the tuna, apple, yogurt, and mustard.

2. Evenly divide the tuna salad among the whole-grain bread to make sandwiches.

SWAP IT: For a sweeter tuna salad, add a drizzle of honey and some dried cranberries. Or for a more savory flavor, add diced scallions and a pinch of salt.

Soy-Glazed Seared Salmon

SERVES: 4 **PREP TIME**: 10 minutes / **COOK TIME**: 15 minutes

30 MINUTES OR LESS | DAIRY-FREE | GLUTEN-FREE

Whether you already enjoy salmon or are just learning to appreciate this omega-3-rich fish, Soy-Glazed Seared Salmon is one of the best recipes to have in your repertoire because it uses ingredients that you likely already have. I recommend using a flexible spatula when cooking fish, as it makes it easier to flip the more delicate protein, but a regular silicone spatula will work, as well.

6 tablespoons low-sodium soy sauce, gluten-free if needed

2 tablespoons rice vinegar

3 garlic cloves, minced

⅛ teaspoon ground ginger, or 4 teaspoons grated fresh ginger

2 teaspoons honey

½ teaspoon red pepper flakes

4 (6-ounce) salmon fillets, skin-on

4 teaspoons extra-virgin olive oil

2 scallions, sliced, for garnish (optional)

Per serving: Calories: 426; Total fat: 25g; Saturated fat: 3g; Cholesterol: 0mg; Sodium: 929mg; Carbohydrates: 5g; Fiber: 0g; Sugar: 3g; Protein: 45g

1. Preheat the oven to 425°F. On the stovetop, preheat a large cast-iron skillet or other oven-safe skillet on high heat for 10 minutes.

2. In a small saucepan over medium-high heat, bring the soy sauce, vinegar, garlic, and ginger to a simmer and cook for 4 minutes. Remove from the heat and stir in the honey and red pepper flakes. Spoon ¼ cup of the glaze into a small bowl and set aside.

3. Drizzle the salmon with the olive oil. Place the fillets skin-side up in the preheated skillet. Cook for 3 minutes, or until the salmon forms a nice crust. The sides should also turn opaque. Carefully flip the salmon fillets and spoon the cooked glaze over the top of each fillet. Place the skillet in the oven and cook for 6 minutes. The salmon should still look a bit under-cooked in the center. Remove the pan from the oven and cover with foil. Let rest for 4 minutes.

4. Serve with the reserved glaze and garnished with scallions (if using).

SWAP IT: If you can't find gluten-free soy sauce, use low-sodium tamari instead. You can also use coconut aminos, which are also gluten-free and generally lower in sodium than soy sauce.

Baked Salmon Patties over Simple Arugula Salad

SERVES 4 **PREP TIME**: 10 minutes / **COOK TIME**: 20 minutes

30 MINUTES OR LESS | DAIRY-FREE

Canned salmon is a less expensive way to get a serving of omega-3-rich fish during the week. These salmon patties require just a handful of pantry staples for a meal that's flavorful and healthy. They also make a great appetizer. Simply make eight small patties instead of four large ones and reduce the cooking time to 8 minutes, or until the patties are golden brown on both sides.

For the salmon patties

1 (15-ounce)
can wild-caught
salmon, drained

2 large eggs, beaten

½ cup whole-grain
bread crumbs

¾ teaspoon salt

½ teaspoon garlic powder

¼ cup chopped fresh
parsley or dill

1 tablespoon freshly
squeezed lemon juice

2 teaspoons extra-virgin
olive oil

For the salad

4 teaspoons extra-virgin
olive oil

4 teaspoons freshly
squeezed lemon juice

Pinch freshly ground
black pepper

To make the salmon patties

1. Preheat the oven to 425°F. Line a large baking sheet with parchment paper.

2. In a large bowl, combine the salmon, eggs, bread crumbs, salt, garlic powder, parsley, and lemon juice. Form the mixture into four equal-size patties.

3. Place the patties on the prepared baking sheet and brush the tops with the olive oil. Bake for 10 minutes, flip, and cook for another 5 to 7 minutes. The patties should be golden brown on both sides. Remove from the oven and set aside.

To make the salad

4. While the patties are cooking, make the salad. In a small bowl, whisk together the olive oil, lemon juice, and black pepper. Set the dressing aside.

6 cups baby arugula, rinsed and dried

Plain low-fat Greek yogurt, for serving (optional)

Per serving: Calories: 289; Total fat: 14g; Saturated fat: 3g; Cholesterol: 126mg; Sodium: 676mg; Carbohydrates: 12g; Fiber: 3g; Sugar: 1g; Protein: 29g

5. Divide the arugula among four plates. Drizzle the dressing evenly over the arugula and top each salad with a cooked salmon patty. Top with a dollop of Greek yogurt (if using) and enjoy immediately.

SWAP IT: If you already have salmon fillets at home, you can use 1 pound of cooked salmon instead of canned. For a flavor twist, use 2 teaspoons of Old Bay seasoning instead of the salt and garlic powder.

Baked Pesto Salmon

SERVES 4 **PREP TIME**: 10 minutes / **COOK TIME**: 15 minutes

5-INGREDIENT | 30 MINUTES OR LESS | DAIRY-FREE | GLUTEN-FREE | ONE-PAN

This Baked Pesto Salmon is a rich yet nutrient-packed dinner. Although easy enough for a weeknight meal, it also makes an impressive dish for a dinner party. To make this recipe even faster, make the Vegan Spinach Pesto the day before. Serve this salmon recipe over whole-grain pasta or brown rice with a side of roasted vegetables.

Nonstick cooking spray, for greasing the pan

4 (6-ounce) salmon fillets

Salt

Freshly ground black pepper

3 tablespoons extra-virgin olive oil

¼ cup white wine

2 tablespoons freshly squeezed lemon juice

¼ cup Vegan Spinach Pesto (page 144)

Per serving: Calories: 516; Total fat: 37g; Saturated fat: 5g; Cholesterol: 0mg; Sodium: 154mg; Carbohydrates: 2g; Fiber: 1g; Sugar: 1g; Protein: 44g

1. Preheat the oven to 350°F. Lightly grease a 9-by-13-inch baking dish with nonstick cooking spray.

2. Place the salmon fillets in the prepared baking dish and season with salt and pepper.

3. In a small bowl, whisk together the olive oil, wine, and lemon juice. Pour the mixture over the salmon fillets. Place the salmon in the oven and cook for 12 to 15 minutes, or until it's cooked through and flakes easily with a fork.

4. Remove the salmon from the oven. Evenly distribute the pesto over the fillets. Using the back of a spoon, spread the pesto over the top of each fillet and serve immediately.

SWAP IT: If you don't have white wine or would prefer not to use it, substitute an equal amount of chicken broth or vegetable broth.

Baked Halibut with Tomatoes

SERVES 4 **PREP TIME**: 10 minutes / **COOK TIME**: 15 minutes

30 MINUTES OR LESS | DAIRY-FREE | GLUTEN-FREE | ONE-POT

If you're new to cooking fish, this is a great recipe to start with. Not only is it made in one pan, but covering the fish with tomato sauce as it bakes also results in a juicy, flavorful, foolproof dish. This recipe uses just a handful of Mediterranean-inspired ingredients, so be sure to use fire-roasted diced tomatoes for a deeper, more complex flavor.

1 (15-ounce) can fire-roasted diced tomatoes, drained

2 garlic cloves, minced

2 tablespoons extra-virgin olive oil

½ teaspoon dried oregano

¼ teaspoon salt

¼ teaspoon freshly ground black pepper

½ tablespoon freshly squeezed lemon juice

4 (6-ounce) halibut fillets

Chopped fresh parsley, for garnish (optional)

Capers, for garnish (optional)

Per serving: Calories: 238; Total fat: 9g; Saturated fat: 1g; Cholesterol: 83mg; Sodium: 281mg; Carbohydrates: 5g; Fiber: 1g; Sugar: 3g; Protein: 32g

1. Preheat the oven to 400°F.

2. In a medium bowl, combine the tomatoes, garlic, olive oil, oregano, salt, pepper, and lemon juice. Spread one-third of the tomato mixture in the bottom of a 9-by-13-inch baking dish.

3. Place the halibut fillets on top of the tomato sauce and cover them with the remaining tomato mixture. Bake for 15 minutes, or until the fish is cooked through to an internal temperature of 145°F.

4. Serve immediately, garnished with fresh parsley and capers (if using).

SWAP IT: Any firm-bodied white fish will work. Cod or tilapia in particular would work very well with this dish.

Grilled Fish Tacos with Avocado Crema

SERVES 4 **PREP TIME**: 15 minutes / **COOK TIME**: 10 minutes

30 MINUTES OR LESS | GLUTEN-FREE

Seasoned with lightly spicy Cajun seasoning, these fish tacos have just the right amount of heat, balanced out by a cool and creamy avocado crema. For an added crunch, I recommend serving your tacos with Apple Cider Vinegar Purple Coleslaw. If you like a smokier flavor to your fish tacos, cook the fish on the grill instead of on the stove.

1 large avocado, pitted and peeled

¼ cup low-fat plain Greek yogurt

Juice of 1 small lime

½ teaspoon salt

4 (4-ounce) cod fillets

1 tablespoon Cajun seasoning

1 tablespoon extra-virgin olive oil

8 (6-inch) corn or whole-wheat flour tortillas

Apple Cider Vinegar Purple Coleslaw (page 57), for serving (optional)

1 small lime, cut in quarters, for serving (optional)

Per serving: Calories: 555; Total fat: 19g; Saturated fat: 3g; Cholesterol: 51mg; Sodium: 1763mg; Carbohydrates: 61g; Fiber: 8g; Sugar: 3g; Protein: 32g

1. In a food processor, make the avocado crema by pulsing the avocado, Greek yogurt, lime juice, and salt until the mixture is smooth and creamy. Taste and add more salt as needed. Set aside.

2. Place the cod fillets on a plate or cutting board and rub the Cajun seasoning evenly over each fillet.

3. In a large skillet, heat the oil over medium-high heat. Add the cod fillets and cook for 4 minutes on each side, or until the fish is just opaque and lightly charred. Cut the fillets into 1-inch pieces.

4. Evenly divide the cooked fish among the tortillas. Top each taco with avocado crema and coleslaw (if using) and serve with lime wedges on the side (if using).

SWAP IT: If you don't have Cajun seasoning, combine 1 teaspoon of smoked paprika, 1 teaspoon of garlic powder, ½ teaspoon of chili powder, ½ teaspoon of ground cumin, ¼ teaspoon of salt, and a pinch of black pepper.

Fish en Papillote with Summer Squash

SERVES 4 **PREP TIME**: 15 minutes / **COOK TIME**: 15 minutes

30 MINUTES OR LESS | DAIRY-FREE | GLUTEN-FREE | ONE-POT

En papillote is French for *in paper*. Despite its fancy name, this is actually a very easy and convenient way of cooking fish. Plus, there's very little cleanup. Although the recipe calls for cod fillets, any firm-bodied fish should work, such as halibut, trout, flounder, and even salmon. For extra flavor, serve this recipe with a drizzle of Fresh Herb Chimichurri (page 143).

3 tablespoons extra-virgin olive oil

2 garlic cloves, minced

2 tablespoons chopped fresh parsley

1 small shallot, minced

½ teaspoon salt

¼ teaspoon freshly ground black pepper

1 large lemon, zested and cut into 8 slices

2 medium zucchini, thinly sliced and quartered

2 medium yellow summer squash, thinly sliced and quartered

4 (6-ounce) cod fillets

Per serving: Calories: 286; Total fat: 12g; Saturated fat: 2g; Cholesterol: 75mg; Sodium: 399mg; Carbohydrates: 12g; Fiber: 3g; Sugar: 7g; Protein: 33g

1. Preheat the oven to 425°F.

2. In a small bowl, whisk together the olive oil, garlic, parsley, shallot, salt, pepper, and lemon zest.

3. Cut four squares of parchment paper, each about 12 inches. Lay each square on the countertop. Divide the zucchini and summer squash slices among the four parchment squares, then place the cod fillets on top of the squash. Spoon the olive oil mixture over the fillets and place 2 lemon slices on top of each piece of fish.

4. Fold the parchment packets by lifting the right and left sides of parchment up and toward the center. Touch the two sides together and tightly roll them, folding the other sides in until you reach the fish. Tuck the ends under the packets and place the packets on a large baking sheet so that the ends are held in place between the fish packets and the baking sheet.

5. Roast for 12 to 15 minutes, or until the fish is cooked through and reaches an internal temperature of 145°F. Serve immediately.

MAKE IT EASIER: Prep these packets ahead of time. The vegetables can be cut the day before and the packets can be assembled up to 4 hours before cooking. Just store them in the refrigerator until dinner time.

Fresh Shrimp Summer Rolls

SERVES 4 **PREP TIME**: 20 minutes

5-INGREDIENT | 30 MINUTES OR LESS | DAIRY-FREE | GLUTEN-FREE | NO-COOK

Summer rolls are a traditional Vietnamese appetizer made by wrapping fresh vegetables and various types of proteins in rice paper wrappers. Rice paper wrappers typically come in thin, round packages and are found in the international foods aisle of most large supermarkets. You can also buy them online. This is one of my favorite meals for getting the whole family involved; you can set out all the ingredients on a counter and have each family member assemble their own rolls. For extra flavor, I recommend adding fresh mint and basil leaves to your spring rolls.

12 (6-inch) rice paper wrappers

6 large green lettuce leaves, cut in half

2 medium carrots, peeled and cut into matchsticks

1 large avocado, sliced

1 pound cooked shrimp, shells and tails removed, sliced in half

Family-Favorite Peanut Sauce (page 141), for serving (optional)

Per serving: Calories: 286; Total fat: 6g; Saturated fat: 1g; Cholesterol: 214mg; Sodium: 187mg; Carbohydrates: 27g; Fiber: 4g; Sugar: 3g; Protein: 32g

1. Fill a large, shallow dish, such as a 9-inch baking pan, with warm water. Working one at a time, submerge one of the rice paper wrappers into the warm water for 15 seconds. The rice paper should be soft and pliable but still slightly firm. Immediately remove the wrapper from the water and place it on a large cutting board.

2. Place one lettuce leaf half in the middle of the wrapper. Add a few carrot sticks, a slice or two of avocado, and some shrimp on top of the lettuce. Roll up the summer roll by gently pulling one side of the wrapper over the filling. Start rolling, as you would with a burrito, tucking in the sides and filling as you go. You want a very tight roll. Set the assembled summer roll aside seam-side down. Repeat with the remaining rice paper wrappers.

3. When all the summer rolls are assembled, slice each roll in half and serve with peanut sauce (if using).

SWAP IT: To make this recipe vegan, use baked or pan-fried tofu instead of the shrimp. You can also add extra vegetables, such as sliced bell peppers, sliced cucumbers, or shredded cabbage.

Lemon-Garlic Shrimp Skewers

SERVES 6 **PREP TIME**: 15 minutes / **COOK TIME**: 10 minutes

30 MINUTES OR LESS | DAIRY-FREE | GLUTEN-FREE

These Lemon-Garlic Shrimp Skewers are simply seasoned yet so flavorful and juicy! If you want, you can grill them. Simply reduce the cooking time to 3 to 5 minutes, depending on how hot your grill is. You can also place the shrimp and lemon halves in a grill basket, rather than making skewers. Whether you make them in the oven or on the grill, this recipe can be enjoyed year-round. I recommend serving these skewers with the Strawberry and Avocado Salad (page 54).

Nonstick cooking spray, for greasing the pan

1½ pounds uncooked shrimp, peeled and deveined

4 small lemons, sliced into ½-inch slices and halved

Salt

Freshly ground black pepper

¼ cup extra-virgin olive oil

¼ cup freshly squeezed lemon juice

4 garlic cloves, minced

1½ tablespoons Italian seasoning

2 tablespoons chopped fresh parsley (optional)

Per serving: Calories: 191; Total fat: 10g; Saturated fat: 1g; Cholesterol: 183mg; Sodium: 162mg; Carbohydrates: 4g; Fiber: 1g; Sugar: 1g; Protein: 23g

1. Preheat the oven to 425°F. Lightly grease a large baking sheet with nonstick cooking spray.

2. Using metal or wooden skewers, thread the shrimp and lemon slices onto the skewers. Season with salt and pepper. Place the skewers on the prepared baking sheet and bake for 7 to 10 minutes, or until the shrimp are pink. Remove from the oven.

3. In a small bowl, whisk together the olive oil, lemon juice, garlic, Italian seasoning, and parsley (if using). Either brush the garlic sauce over the cooked shrimp skewers or remove the shrimp from the skewers and toss them with the garlic sauce in a large serving bowl. Serve immediately.

SWAP IT: You can use scallops in place of the shrimp. Simply increase the cooking time to 11 to 14 minutes.

Shrimp Quinoa Fried "Rice"

SERVES 4 **PREP TIME**: 10 minutes / **COOK TIME**: 20 minutes

30 MINUTES OR LESS | DAIRY-FREE | GLUTEN-FREE | ONE-POT

This fried "rice" is a healthy twist on a take-out classic. Quinoa is a naturally gluten-free whole grain that's higher in protein, fiber, calcium, and zinc than brown rice. Of course, if you have another leftover grain, feel free to use it instead of the quinoa. To get the texture of this fried "rice" just right, I like to make the quinoa a day or two ahead of time.

2 tablespoons plus 1 teaspoon extra-virgin olive oil, divided

2 large eggs, beaten

1 pound uncooked shrimp, peeled and deveined

2 garlic cloves, minced

3 scallions, sliced, white and green parts separated

2 large carrots, peeled and diced

½ cup frozen peas

½ cup frozen corn

3 tablespoons low-sodium soy sauce, gluten-free if needed

3 cups cooked quinoa

Red pepper flakes (optional)

Per serving: Calories: 413; Total fat: 13g; Saturated fat: 2g; Cholesterol: 265mg; Sodium: 672mg; Carbohydrates: 41g; Fiber: 7g; Sugar: 6g; Protein: 35g

1. In a large wok or skillet, heat 1 teaspoon of oil over medium-low heat. Add the eggs and stir frequently to scramble them. Cook until the eggs are just about set, about 4 minutes. Remove the cooked eggs to a plate and set aside.

2. Increase the heat to medium-high and add 1 tablespoon of olive oil. When the oil is hot, add the shrimp. Cook for 2 to 3 minutes, stirring occasionally, until the shrimp are opaque and pink. Remove the shrimp to the same plate as the eggs and set aside.

3. Add the remaining 1 tablespoon of olive oil, the garlic, and the white parts of the scallions to the skillet. Cook for 1 to 2 minutes, or until the garlic is fragrant. Add the carrots, peas, and corn. Stir frequently until the vegetables are heated through and the carrots are slightly tender, about 5 minutes.

4. Add the soy sauce and quinoa to the skillet. Stir to combine and cook for 3 minutes, or until the quinoa is heated through. Add the cooked eggs and shrimp back to the skillet and stir to combine.

5. Garnish with the scallion greens and red pepper flakes (if using) and serve immediately.

MAKE IT EASIER: To make this dish even easier, use frozen carrots instead of fresh. You can also buy microwavable quinoa or brown rice to save even more time.

Pan-Seared Scallops with Zucchini Noodles

SERVES 4 **PREP TIME**: 10 minutes / **COOK TIME**: 10 minutes

30 MINUTES OR LESS | DAIRY-FREE | GLUTEN-FREE | ONE-POT

These savory scallops in a velvety citrus sauce are the perfect date-night meal. To help balance out the dish, the scallops and sauce are served over a bed of fresh spiralized zucchini noodles. If you can't get fresh scallops, buy frozen scallops and thaw them in the refrigerator the night before making this dish.

4 medium zucchini, spiralized and patted dry

Salt

2 tablespoons extra-virgin olive oil

1½ pounds sea scallops

Zest and juice of 1 large orange

Juice of 1 medium lemon

1 tablespoon grated fresh ginger

2 tablespoons coconut milk

Per serving: Calories: 182; Total fat: 8g; Saturated fat: 1g; Cholesterol: 30mg; Sodium: 207mg; Carbohydrates: 13g; Fiber: 3g; Sugar: 8g; Protein: 17g

1. In a large skillet over medium-high heat, sauté the zucchini with a pinch of salt for 2 to 3 minutes, or until the zucchini is heated through but not too soft. Remove from the skillet and set aside.

2. Add the olive oil to the skillet. When the oil is hot, place the scallops in the pan, leaving some room between each scallop to help them cook more evenly. Sprinkle them with another pinch of salt and cook for 90 seconds to 2 minutes. Flip and cook for another 90 seconds, or until they're lightly seared on both sides. Remove the scallops from the pan and set aside.

3. Reduce the heat to medium and add the orange zest and juice, lemon juice, ginger, and coconut milk. Whisk continuously until the sauce comes to a light simmer, about 2 minutes. Add the scallops back into the pan and spoon the sauce over the top.

4. Divide the zucchini noodles among four bowls and add the scallops and sauce on top.

MAKE IT EASIER: If you don't have a spiralizer, you can buy pre-spiralized zucchini noodles at the store, or you can make zucchini ribbons instead by using a vegetable peeler.

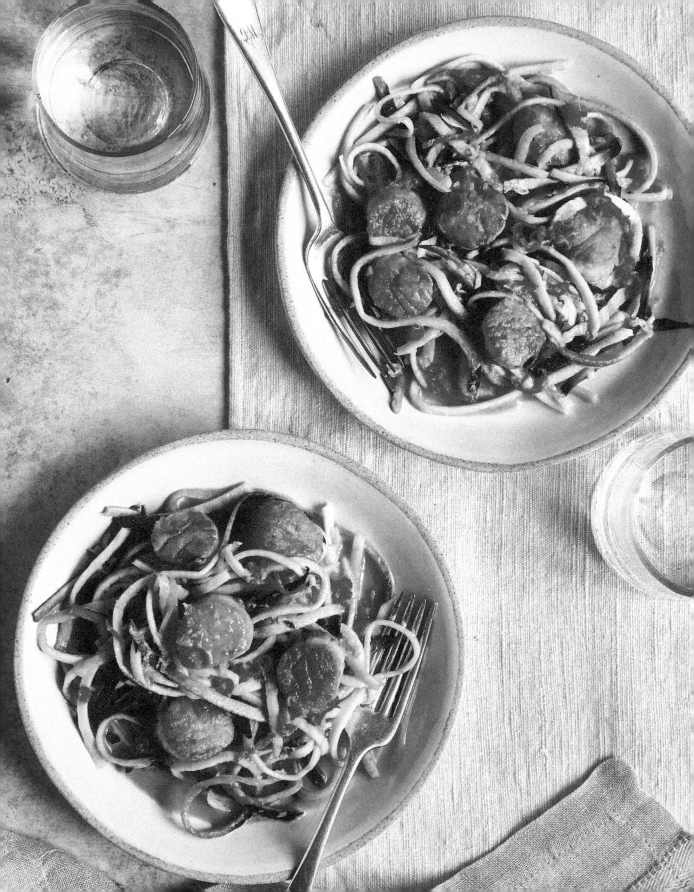

Shrimp and Scallop Paella

SERVES 6 **PREP TIME**: 10 minutes / **COOK TIME**: 30 minutes

DAIRY-FREE | GLUTEN-FREE | ONE-PAN

Paella is a Spanish rice dish that's traditionally cooked over an open fire. Although this recipe is made on the stove, it still retains many of the original flavors, including saffron. This recipe calls for Arborio rice instead. If you want to use the more traditional bomba rice, note that you may need to adjust the amount of broth based on the instructions on the package.

2 tablespoons extra-virgin olive oil

1 large shallot, diced

4 garlic cloves, minced

2 tablespoons tomato paste

1 teaspoon smoked paprika

1 teaspoon saffron threads

¾ teaspoon salt

1½ cups uncooked Arborio rice

5 ounces fresh baby spinach, roughly chopped

3 cups low-sodium chicken broth

1 pound uncooked shrimp, peeled and deveined

½ pound sea scallops

Per serving: Calories: 338; Total fat: 6g; Saturated fat: 1g; Cholesterol: 132mg; Sodium: 493mg; Carbohydrates: 45g; Fiber: 3g; Sugar: 2g; Protein: 28g

1. In a large skillet, heat the oil over medium heat. Add the shallot and garlic and sauté for 2 minutes, or until fragrant. Add the tomato paste, paprika, saffron, and salt. Cook until the tomato paste is fully mixed in, about 2 minutes. Add the rice and cook for 3 minutes, stirring frequently.

2. Stir in the spinach and broth. Bring to a simmer. Reduce the heat to low and simmer, uncovered, for 10 minutes, or until the rice is soft but still chewy.

3. Add the shrimp and scallops to the pan, pressing them down into the rice so that they're almost covered with the remaining liquid. Cook for 10 minutes, or until the liquid has been fully absorbed and the shrimp and scallops are cooked through. Serve immediately.

SWAP IT: Feel free to use clams or mussels instead of the scallops. You can also add additional vegetables, such as peas, diced carrots, green beans, or asparagus.

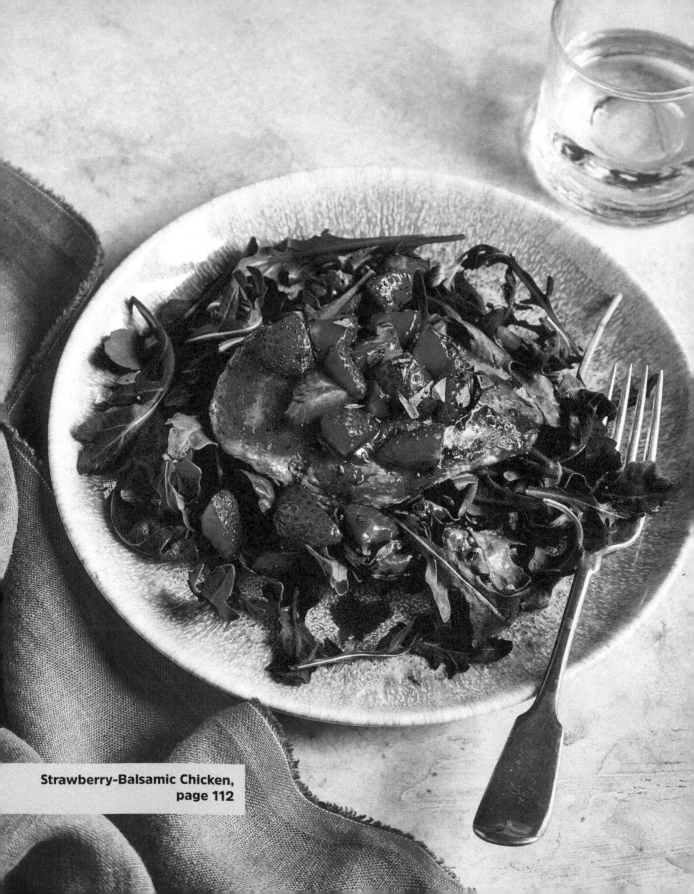

Strawberry-Balsamic Chicken, page 112

CHAPTER 7

Poultry and Meat Mains

Spiced Chicken Pita Wraps

SERVES 4 **PREP TIME**: 15 minutes / **COOK TIME**: 10 minutes

30 MINUTES OR LESS | DAIRY-FREE

Chicken thighs are my go-to protein when I need to cook chicken quickly over high heat. Because they're a bit higher in fat than chicken breasts, they're less likely to dry out. These wraps are easily customizable, depending on what spices you have in your cabinet. If you have the time, I recommend serving these with Simple Tzatziki (page 142).

1 pound boneless, skinless chicken thighs, cut into ½-inch cubes

1 teaspoon ground cumin

1 teaspoon smoked paprika

¼ teaspoon ground turmeric

1 teaspoon salt

1 tablespoon extra-virgin olive oil

4 large green lettuce leaves

1 large cucumber, sliced

2 large Roma tomatoes, sliced

8 tablespoons hummus

4 medium whole-wheat pita breads

Per serving: Calories: 397; Total fat: 14g; Saturated fat: 1g; Cholesterol: 91mg; Sodium: 1135mg; Carbohydrates: 45g; Fiber: 8g; Sugar: 7g; Protein: 28g

1. In a large bowl, combine the chicken, cumin, paprika, turmeric, and salt. Set aside.

2. In a large skillet, heat the oil over medium high heat. Add the chicken in a single layer. Cook for 4 minutes, or until the bottoms of the chicken pieces are lightly browned. Flip the chicken and cook for another 3 to 4 minutes, or until the chicken is browned and cooked through. Set aside.

3. Assemble the wraps by evenly dividing the chicken, lettuce, cucumber, tomato, and hummus among the pitas.

SWAP IT: This recipe also works well as a salad. Instead of wrapping the chicken and vegetables in the pita bread, simply place them over a bed of green lettuce or spinach. I still recommend topping the dish with hummus and tzatziki.

Oatmeal-Crusted Baked Chicken Cutlets

SERVES 4 **PREP TIME**: 10 minutes / **COOK TIME**: 25 minutes

5-INGREDIENT | DAIRY-FREE | GLUTEN-FREE

Here's a healthier twist on traditional breaded chicken cutlets, which are often pan-fried rather than baked. This recipe is a great family staple, and it can be paired with a wide variety of side dishes. In the warmer months, it goes well with the Strawberry and Avocado Salad (page 54), and in the colder months, you can pair it with the Go-To Sautéed Garlic Kale (page 67) and some mashed sweet potatoes.

1½ cups rolled old-fashioned oats, gluten-free if needed, pulsed into a coarse flour

1 teaspoon paprika

½ teaspoon salt

2 large eggs, beaten

4 (4-ounce) boneless, skinless chicken breasts, patted dry with a paper towel

Per serving: Calories: 172; Total fat: 5g; Saturated fat: 1g; Cholesterol: 165mg; Sodium: 373mg; Carbohydrates: 1g; Fiber: 0g; Sugar: 0g; Protein: 28g

1. Preheat the oven to 400°F. Line a large baking sheet with parchment paper.

2. In a shallow bowl, combine the pulsed oats, paprika, and salt. Set aside. In another shallow bowl, add the beaten eggs.

3. Working one at a time, dip each chicken cutlet into the egg mixture. Allow some of the egg to drip off before dredging the cutlet in the oat mixture, pressing down to fully coat. Place the breaded chicken cutlet on the prepared baking sheet and repeat with the remaining chicken cutlets.

4. Roast the cutlets for 10 minutes. Flip the chicken over and cook for another 10 to 12 minutes, or until the chicken is cooked through to an internal temperature of 165°F. Serve immediately.

SWAP IT: For slightly spicy chicken, add ¼ to ½ teaspoon of cayenne pepper to the oat mix. You can also add 1 teaspoon of Italian seasoning for a different flavor profile.

Strawberry-Balsamic Chicken

SERVES 4 **PREP TIME**: 10 minutes / **COOK TIME**: 15 minutes

30 MINUTES OR LESS | DAIRY-FREE | GLUTEN-FREE

This is the ultimate summer meal. After cooking the chicken breasts on the stove, you'll top them with a slightly sweet strawberry-basil balsamic relish for an addictive sweet and savory flavor combination. This chicken dish is great over a simple bed of arugula, or it can be served on top of a whole grain, such as farro or quinoa.

6 tablespoons balsamic vinegar

Salt

2 cups chopped fresh strawberries

1 cup chopped fresh basil

2 tablespoons extra-virgin olive oil

2 garlic cloves, crushed

4 (4-ounce) boneless, skinless chicken breasts, pounded to 1-inch thickness

Freshly ground black pepper

Per serving: Calories: 246; Total fat: 10g; Saturated fat: 2g; Cholesterol: 83mg; Sodium: 392mg; Carbohydrates: 11g; Fiber: 2g; Sugar: 7g; Protein: 27g

1. In a small pot over medium-high heat, combine the balsamic vinegar and a pinch of salt. Bring to a boil, then reduce the heat to medium-low. Simmer for 10 minutes, or until it's reduced by half. Remove the pot from the heat and stir in the strawberries and basil. Set aside.

2. Meanwhile, in a large skillet, heat the oil over medium heat. Add the garlic and cook for 1 to 2 minutes, or until fragrant. Add the chicken breasts and season with salt and pepper. Cook for 5 minutes, or until the bottom of each breast is golden brown. Flip and cook for another 3 to 5 minutes, or until the chicken is cooked through to an internal temperature of 165°F.

3. To serve, place one cooked chicken breast on each plate and spoon on the strawberry-balsamic topping.

SWAP IT: You can also serve the strawberry-balsamic glaze over roasted or grilled salmon. Delicious!

Sheet-Pan Chicken Fajitas

SERVES 4 **PREP TIME**: 15 minutes / **COOK TIME**: 25 minutes

DAIRY-FREE | GLUTEN-FREE | ONE-PAN

Chicken fajitas are an easy family meal, as each person can customize their own with different toppings and sides. By having the chicken and vegetables cook in one pan, this recipe makes dinnertime even easier! While the recipe calls for onions and bell peppers, feel free to switch up the vegetables.

1 pound boneless, skinless chicken breasts, sliced into thin strips

½ large yellow onion, thinly sliced

3 bell peppers, seeded and thinly sliced

1½ tablespoons extra-virgin olive oil

2 tablespoons freshly squeezed lime juice

1½ teaspoons chili powder

¾ teaspoon paprika

¾ teaspoon ground cumin

¾ teaspoon garlic powder

½ teaspoon salt

¼ teaspoon freshly ground black pepper

12 small corn or whole-wheat flour tortillas

Guacamole, for serving

Salsa, for serving

Per serving: Calories: 469; Total fat: 16g; Saturated fat: 1g; Cholesterol: 83mg; Sodium: 1191mg; Carbohydrates: 47g; Fiber: 18g; Sugar: 6g; Protein: 48g

1. Preheat the oven to 400°F. Line a large baking sheet with parchment paper.

2. In a large bowl, combine the chicken, onion, bell peppers, olive oil, lime juice, chili powder, paprika, cumin, garlic powder, salt, and pepper. Toss well to coat the chicken and vegetables in the seasoning.

3. Pour the mixture onto the prepared baking sheet. Spread out the chicken and vegetables in a single layer on the pan. Bake for 20 minutes, stirring halfway through. Then set the oven to broil and broil on high for 2 to 3 minutes, or until the vegetables are lightly charred.

4. Serve the chicken and vegetables with the tortillas and the guacamole and salsa.

SWAP IT: If you don't have all the spices, you can use a packet of fajita seasoning instead. Just make sure to look for a low-sodium blend.

Light and Lemony Chicken Piccata

SERVES 4 **PREP TIME**: 10 minutes / **COOK TIME**: 20 minutes

30 MINUTES OR LESS | DAIRY-FREE | ONE-POT

Chicken piccata is an Italian dish that typically involves dredging thin chicken cutlets in flour and coating them in a sauce made from lemon juice, butter, white wine, and capers. This recipe is a lightened-up version that uses olive oil in place of butter, meaning less fat overall. Serve it with whole-grain pasta and sautéed vegetables for a balanced dinner.

¼ cup white whole-wheat flour

½ teaspoon salt

½ teaspoon freshly ground black pepper

1 pound bone-in skinless chicken breasts, pounded to ¼-inch thickness and cut into 8 cutlets

2 tablespoons extra-virgin olive oil, divided

1 large shallot, diced

1 garlic clove, minced

1 cup low-sodium chicken broth

¼ cup dry white wine

2 tablespoons freshly squeezed lemon juice

2 cups roughly chopped fresh baby spinach

Lemon slices, for serving (optional)

Drained capers, for serving (optional)

Chopped fresh parsley, for serving (optional)

1. In a shallow bowl or plate, whisk together the flour, salt, and pepper. Dredge each chicken cutlet in the flour mixture, turning to coat, and place the coated chicken on a cutting board or large plate. Reserve the flour mixture to thicken the sauce later.

2. In a large skillet, heat 2 teaspoons of oil over medium-high heat. Add four of the chicken cutlets to the pan and cook for 3 to 4 minutes, or until the bottom is lightly browned. Flip the chicken and cook for another 2 to 3 minutes, or until lightly browned. Remove the chicken to a plate. Add another 2 teaspoons of oil to the skillet and repeat the cooking process with the remaining chicken. Transfer the cooked chicken to the plate.

3. Add the remaining 2 teaspoons of oil to the pan and increase the heat to medium-high. Add the shallots and garlic. Cook for 2 minutes, or until fragrant.

4. Add the leftover dredging flour to the pan and stir in the broth, wine, and lemon juice. Bring the mixture to a simmer, stirring constantly. Add the spinach and chicken cutlets to the pan. Using a spoon, coat the chicken cutlets with the sauce. Simmer for 3 to 4 minutes, or until the sauce has thickened and the chicken is fully cooked.

Per serving: Calories: 286; Total fat: 10g; Saturated fat: 2g; Cholesterol: 83mg; Sodium: 397mg; Carbohydrates: 11g; Fiber: 2g; Sugar: 2g; Protein: 28g

5. Serve with lemon slices, capers, and fresh parsley (if using).

SWAP IT: If you don't want to buy a bottle of wine just to make this dish, you can use another ½ cup of chicken broth instead.

One-Pan Turmeric Chicken

SERVES 6 **PREP TIME**: 10 minutes / **COOK TIME**: 30 minutes

DAIRY-FREE | GLUTEN-FREE | ONE-PAN

A staple in Indian cuisine, turmeric is a spice that also contains compounds that have been shown to have potent anti-inflammatory and antioxidant effects. A handful of other spices provide a rich, complex flavor to this otherwise simple dish. Store leftovers in an airtight container in the refrigerator for up to 4 days.

1 tablespoon extra-virgin olive oil

1½ teaspoons ground turmeric

Pinch freshly ground black pepper

6 boneless, skinless chicken thighs

2 garlic cloves, grated

2 medium plum tomatoes, chopped

2 medium carrots, diced

4 cups roughly chopped fresh baby spinach

3 scallions, sliced, white and green parts separated

2 teaspoons yellow curry powder

½ teaspoon cinnamon

½ teaspoon ground cumin

1 cup uncooked basmati rice

1. In a deep sauté pan or cast-iron skillet, heat the oil over medium-high heat until it's hot and shimmering. Add the turmeric, pepper, and chicken thighs. Cook until the thighs are browned, about 4 minutes. Flip and cook for another 4 minutes, or until the bottoms are browned. Remove the thighs from the pan and place on a paper towel–lined plate.

2. Reduce the heat to medium and add the garlic, tomatoes, carrots, spinach, white parts of the scallions, curry powder, cinnamon, and cumin. Cook for 2 minutes, stirring frequently, until the spices are fragrant and the carrots are just starting to brown.

3. Add the rice to the pan and cook for 1 minute. Place the chicken thighs on top of the rice. Pour the broth and soy sauce over the chicken. Increase the heat to medium-high and bring the liquid to a boil. Reduce the heat to a low simmer and cover.

2 cups low-sodium
chicken broth

1 tablespoon low-sodium
soy sauce, gluten-free
if needed

Salt

Per serving: Calories: 251;
Total fat: 3g; Saturated fat: 0g;
Cholesterol: 70mg; Sodium:
271mg; Carbohydrates: 32g;
Fiber: 2g; Sugar: 3g; Pro-
tein: 21g

4. Cook for 30 to 35 minutes, or until the rice is cooked
through. Season with salt. Garnish with the green
scallion slices and serve.

MAKE IT EASIER: Heavy-bottomed pans, like a cast-iron
skillet or Dutch oven, tend to absorb and distribute heat
better than regular pans. Although not essential, if you do
have a heavy-bottomed pan, I'd recommend using it for
this recipe.

Spinach-Turkey Meatballs

SERVES 4 **PREP TIME**: 10 minutes / **COOK TIME**: 20 minutes

5-INGREDIENT | 30 MINUTES OR LESS | DAIRY-FREE | GLUTEN-FREE

Whether you have picky kids at home or are simply looking for inspiration, these Spinach-Turkey Meatballs are an easy way to add more leafy greens into your family's diets. For a balanced meal, I recommend serving them with Hidden Veggie Marinara Sauce (page 145) and whole-grain spaghetti. You can also use them to make healthier meatball sub sandwiches. Store leftovers in an airtight container in the refrigerator for up to 4 days.

¼ cup old-fashioned rolled oats, gluten-free if needed, pulsed into a coarse flour

5 ounces fresh baby spinach, finely chopped

½ teaspoon Italian seasoning

Pinch salt

Pinch freshly ground black pepper

1 large egg, lightly beaten

1 pound 93-percent lean ground turkey

Per serving: Calories: 286; Total fat: 15g; Saturated fat: 4g; Cholesterol: 159mg; Sodium: 183mg; Carbohydrates: 5g; Fiber: 1g; Sugar: 0g; Protein: 34g

1. Preheat the oven to 400°F.

2. In a large bowl, combine the pulsed oats, spinach, Italian seasoning, salt, and pepper. Add the egg and ground turkey. Using your hands, mix the ingredients until just combined. You don't want to overwork the turkey.

3. Roll the mixture into golf ball–size meatballs. You should get about 20. Place the meatballs in a 9-by-13-inch baking pan and bake for 20 minutes, or until they're cooked to an internal temperature of 165°F.

4. Remove the meatballs from the pan and toss them in whatever sauce you like.

MAKE IT EASIER: Since you already have a food processor out to pulse the oats, I recommend chopping your spinach using the food processor, as well. If you don't have a food processor, you can use whole-grain bread crumbs instead of the oats.

Juicy Greek Turkey Burgers

SERVES 4 **PREP TIME**: 15 minutes / **COOK TIME**: 10 minutes

30 MINUTES OR LESS | DAIRY-FREE | ONE-PAN

Blended with sun-dried tomatoes and chopped baby spinach, these burgers prove that turkey burgers can be just as flavorful as their beef counterparts. Although any toppings will work, I recommend adding sliced avocado and Simple Tzatziki (page 142). Store leftover cooked turkey burgers in an airtight container in the refrigerator for up to 3 days.

1 pound 93-percent lean ground turkey

¼ cup sun-dried tomatoes, drained and roughly chopped

3 cups finely chopped fresh baby spinach

1 garlic clove, minced

½ teaspoon dried oregano

½ teaspoon onion powder

½ teaspoon salt

¼ teaspoon freshly ground black pepper

1 tablespoon whole-wheat bread crumbs

½ tablespoon extra-virgin olive oil

4 whole-wheat burger buns

Per serving: Calories: 416; Total fat: 17g; Saturated fat: 4g; Cholesterol: 118mg; Sodium: 654mg; Carbohydrates: 29g; Fiber: 4g; Sugar: 4g; Protein: 38g

1. In a large bowl, add the turkey, sun-dried tomatoes, spinach, garlic, oregano, onion powder, salt, pepper, and bread crumbs. Using your hands, mix the ingredients until just combined, making sure not to overwork the turkey. Form the mixture into 4 patties.

2. In a large skillet, heat the oil over medium-high heat. Cook the patties for 5 minutes on each side, or until the outsides are lightly browned and the insides reach an internal temperature of 165°F.

3. Remove the patties from the skillet and place them on a cutting board or large plate to rest for 5 minutes before serving. When you're ready to eat, place each patty on a whole-wheat bun and add any toppings you like.

MAKE IT EASIER: These patties can easily be made a day ahead of time, so all you have to do is cook them when you're ready. Store the formed patties in an airtight container in the refrigerator overnight. Depending on the size of your container, you may want to place a piece of wax or parchment paper between each stacked patty to prevent them from sticking.

Roasted Turkey Tenderloin with Balsamic-Blueberry Sauce

SERVES 4 **PREP TIME**: 10 minutes / **COOK TIME**: 35 minutes

DAIRY-FREE | GLUTEN-FREE | ONE-PAN

Turkey tenderloins are the boneless, skinless parts of the turkey breast. Although some stores will sell them in the meat case, you can also ask your butcher for the cut. Compared to skin-on turkey breasts, turkey tenderloins cook in about half the time, making them a great option for weeknights. Serve with Massaged Kale Salad (page 56) and cooked whole-grain couscous for a fall-inspired meal.

1 tablespoon extra-virgin olive oil

1 pound turkey tenderloin

¾ teaspoon salt

½ teaspoon freshly ground black pepper

1 large shallot, diced

1 tablespoon chopped fresh rosemary

2 cups fresh blueberries

3 tablespoons balsamic vinegar

Per serving: Calories: 241; Total fat: 4g; Saturated fat: 1g; Cholesterol: 71mg; Sodium: 504mg; Carbohydrates: 22g; Fiber: 3g; Sugar: 14g; Protein: 30g

1. Preheat the oven to 450°F.

2. In a large cast-iron skillet or other oven-safe skillet, heat the oil over high heat. Add the turkey tenderloin and season with the salt and pepper. Cook for 5 minutes, or until the bottom is lightly browned. Flip the tenderloin over and transfer the pan to the oven. Cook for 20 minutes, or until the turkey reaches an internal temperature of 165°F. Transfer the turkey to a plate and let it rest while you make the sauce.

3. Return the skillet to the stove. Over medium heat, cook the shallots and rosemary for 1 minute, or until the shallots are lightly browned but not burning. Add the blueberries and balsamic vinegar and cook for 5 minutes, or until the sauce has thickened.

4. Slice the turkey and divide it among 4 plates. Top each serving with the blueberry-balsamic sauce and enjoy immediately.

SWAP IT: This blueberry-balsamic glaze is also delicious over a pork tenderloin.

Blended Mushroom and Beef Burgers

SERVES 4 **PREP TIME**: 10 minutes / **COOK TIME**: 15 minutes

5-INGREDIENT | 30 MINUTES OR LESS | DAIRY-FREE

One easy way to make the traditional hamburger a little healthier is by mixing lean ground beef with diced mushrooms. Not only do mushrooms add essential vitamins and minerals, but they also increase the volume of the patty without using more red meat. Plus, because they're mixed into the ground beef, even non-mushroom lovers will enjoy these burgers. For extra MIND diet goodness, top your burgers with leafy greens.

1 tablespoon extra-virgin olive oil

½ pound cremini mushrooms, finely diced

¾ teaspoon salt, divided

1 pound 90-percent lean ground beef

4 whole-wheat burger buns

Per serving: Calories: 428; Total fat: 18g; Saturated fat: 5g; Cholesterol: 100mg; Sodium: 738mg; Carbohydrates: 28g; Fiber: 4g; Sugar: 4g; Protein: 39g

1. In a medium skillet, heat the oil over medium-high heat. When the oil is hot, add the diced mushrooms and ¼ teaspoon of salt. Cook for 5 minutes, stirring occasionally, until the mushrooms are lightly browned.

2. In a large bowl, combine the cooked mushrooms and ground beef. Using your hands, mix the mushrooms and beef together to combine, being careful not to overwork the meat. Form the mixture into 4 patties and set aside.

3. Heat a grill or griddle to medium-high heat. Just before adding the burgers to the grill, sprinkle the tops of each burger with the remaining ½ teaspoon of salt. Add the patties to the heated grill and cook for 4 to 5 minutes on each side for medium-rare or 6 to 7 minutes on each side for medium.

4. Remove the burgers from the heat and allow them to rest for 5 minutes. Serve on whole-wheat buns with any toppings you like.

SWAP IT: If it's available at your grocery store, ground bison is a great substitute for ground beef; it's lower in saturated fat and higher in protein.

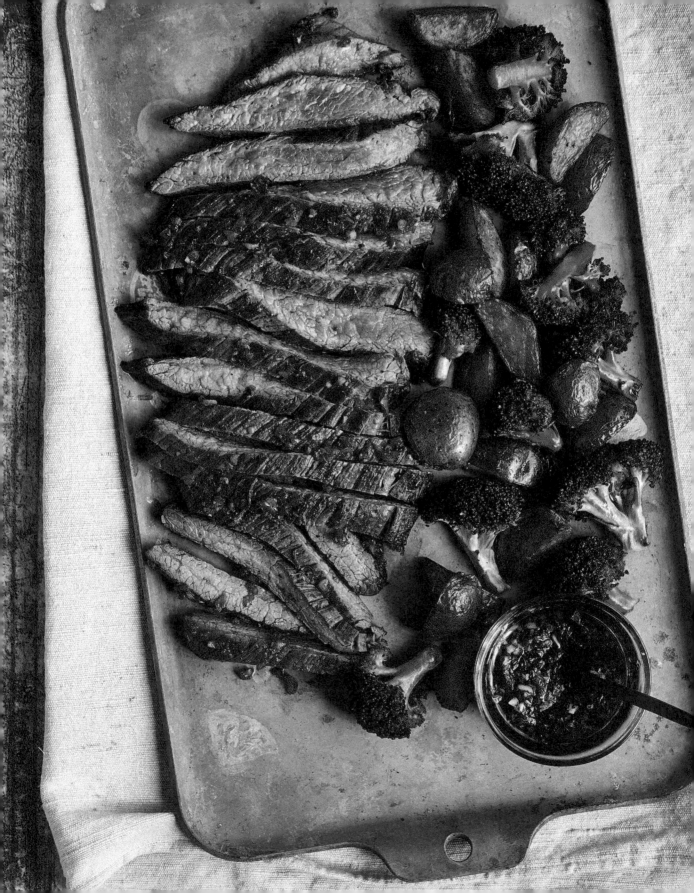

Sheet-Pan Flank Steak and Veggies with Chimichurri

SERVES 6 **PREP TIME**: 10 minutes / **COOK TIME**: 20 minutes

30 MINUTES OR LESS | DAIRY-FREE | GLUTEN-FREE | ONE-PAN

The classic steak and potatoes combo gets a flavorful and healthier twist with this veggie sheet-pan meal. Fresh Herb Chimichurri is what takes this dish over the top. Although this meal is filling enough on its own, you can also pair this recipe with a simple side salad for a serving of leafy greens.

Nonstick cooking spray, for greasing the pan

2 pounds small red potatoes, cut into quarters

2 tablespoons extra-virgin olive oil, divided

4 garlic cloves, minced, divided

Salt

Freshly ground black pepper

1½ pounds flank steak

2 cups broccoli florets

Fresh Herb Chimichurri (page 143)

Per serving: Calories: 373; Total fat: 16g; Saturated fat: 4g; Cholesterol: 78mg; Sodium: 225mg; Carbohydrates: 28g; Fiber: 4g; Sugar: 3g; Protein: 29g

1. Preheat the oven to high broil. Line a large baking sheet with foil and lightly coat it with nonstick cooking spray.

2. Place the potatoes on the prepared baking sheet and drizzle with 1 tablespoon of olive oil and half the minced garlic. Sprinkle the potatoes with salt and pepper and broil for 6 to 8 minutes, or until they are just starting to lightly brown. Remove the pan from the oven.

3. Using a spatula, make space on the pan to add the flank steak and broccoli. Drizzle the remaining 1 tablespoon of olive oil over the broccoli and stir well to coat. Add the remaining garlic on top of the steak and sprinkle the steak and broccoli with salt and pepper.

4. Return the baking sheet to the oven and broil for 5 minutes. Flip the steak and broil for another 5 to 7 minutes, or until the steak is cooked to your desired level of doneness. For a medium-rare steak, the internal temperature should be 130°F to 135°F. For medium, cook your steak to 135°F to 145°F. Remove the pan from the oven and allow the steak to rest for 5 minutes.

Continued ▶

5. Thinly slice the steak and place it on a large serving dish along with the broccoli and potatoes. Drizzle chimichurri over the top and serve immediately.

MAKE IT EASIER: To make this recipe even easier, you can use a store-bought chimichurri or salsa verde.

Fall Harvest Sheet-Pan Pork Tenderloin

SERVES 4 **PREP TIME**: 20 minutes / **COOK TIME**: 25 minutes

DAIRY-FREE | GLUTEN-FREE | ONE-PAN

With a combination of pork, apple, Brussels sprouts, and maple syrup, this sheet-pan meal is packed with fall flavors. Although you may be more familiar with pork chops, I prefer to use a pork tenderloin because it tends to stay juicier when cooked at a high heat. Pair it with the Massaged Kale Salad (page 56) and a cooked whole grain, like farro or quinoa.

1 pound boneless pork tenderloin

3 tablespoons Dijon mustard, divided

1 teaspoon salt, divided

1 teaspoon freshly ground black pepper, divided

1 pound carrots, peeled and sliced into rounds

1 pound Brussels sprouts, outer leaves and ends trimmed, halved

1 large apple, cored and chopped

2 tablespoons pure maple syrup

2 teaspoons extra-virgin olive oil

1 teaspoon dried thyme

Per serving: Calories: 314; Total fat: 8g; Saturated fat: 2g; Cholesterol: 75mg; Sodium: 1023mg; Carbohydrates: 37g; Fiber: 9g; Sugar: 20g; Protein: 30g

1. Preheat the oven to 450°F. Line a large baking sheet with parchment paper.

2. Place the pork tenderloin in the center of the baking sheet. Rub 1 tablespoon of mustard evenly over the top and sides, then sprinkle with ½ teaspoon of salt and ½ teaspoon of pepper.

3. In a large bowl, combine the carrots, Brussels sprouts, apple, remaining 2 tablespoons of mustard, maple syrup, olive oil, thyme, remaining ½ teaspoon salt, and remaining ½ teaspoon pepper. Toss to combine.

4. Transfer the vegetable mixture to the baking sheet and spread it out in a single layer around the pork. Cook for 20 to 25 minutes, turning the baking sheet halfway through, or until the pork reaches an internal temperature of 140°F. Remove the pan from the oven and allow the pork to rest for 5 minutes before slicing. Serve hot.

SWAP IT: If you can't find a pork tenderloin, you can use 1 pound of pork chops instead. Reduce the cooking time to 12 to 16 minutes, or until they're cooked through.

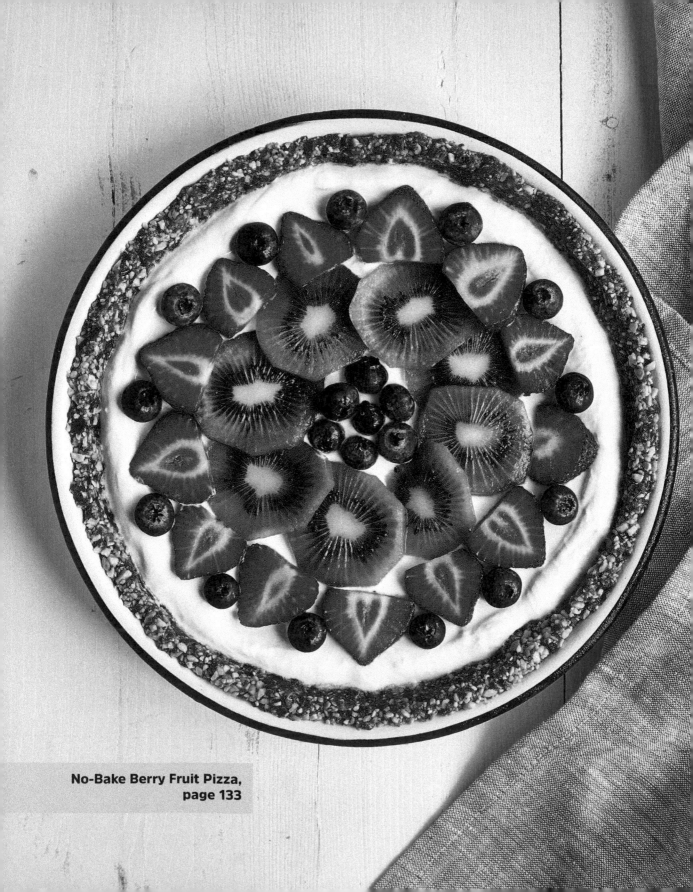

**No-Bake Berry Fruit Pizza,
page 133**

CHAPTER 8

Snacks and Sweet Treats

Superfood Trail Mix

MAKES 2 cups **PREP TIME**: 5 minutes

5-INGREDIENT | 30 MINUTES OR LESS | DAIRY-FREE | GLUTEN-FREE
NO-COOK | VEGAN

Trail mix is the ultimate easy snack. You can mix and match any nuts, seeds, and dried fruits that you have in the pantry. Plus, it has a long shelf life and is perfect to take on the go. This mix is chock-full of MIND diet superfoods: vitamin E–rich almonds, omega-3–rich walnuts, and antioxidant-packed dried blueberries and goji berries. The raw cacao nibs are optional, but they add an extra boost of brain-healthy flavonoids and a deep chocolate flavor. Store this mix in a cool, dry place for up to 6 months.

½ cup roasted almonds

½ cup roasted walnuts

½ cup dried blueberries

¼ cup dried goji berries

¼ cup raw cacao nibs (optional)

Per serving (¼ cup):
Calories: 122; Total fat: 8g; Saturated fat: 1g; Cholesterol: 0mg; Sodium: 4mg; Carbohydrates: 11g; Fiber: 3g; Sugar: 7g; Protein: 3g

In a medium bowl, combine the almonds, walnuts, dried blueberries, dried goji berries, and raw cacao nibs (if using). Store this mix in an airtight container or portion it out into snack-size bags.

SWAP IT: Pecans, dried cranberries, and pumpkin seeds make a great mix for the fall, while dried cherries can add a sharp punch of flavor. Vegan dark chocolate chips can be used in place of the raw cacao nibs.

Rosemary and Sea Salt Roasted Almonds

MAKES 3 cups **PREP TIME**: 10 minutes / **COOK TIME**: 20 minutes

5-INGREDIENT | 30 MINUTES OR LESS | DAIRY-FREE | GLUTEN-FREE
ONE-PAN | VEGAN

Almonds are a MIND diet superfood packed with important nutrients, including vitamin E, manganese, magnesium, fiber, and healthy fats. They're also a good source of protein. Unlike store-bought nuts, homemade roasted almonds give you full control over the type of oil used and the amount of sodium added. You can enjoy these warm, or you can cool them completely and store them in an airtight container for up to 2 weeks in a cool, dry place. You can also store them in the freezer for up to 3 months.

3 cups whole raw almonds

2 tablespoons extra-virgin olive oil

1 teaspoon dried rosemary

¾ teaspoon fine sea salt

Per serving (¼ cup):
Calories: 208; Total fat: 19g; Saturated fat: 2g; Cholesterol: 0mg; Sodium: 148mg; Carbohydrates: 7g; Fiber: 4g; Sugar: 1g; Protein: 7g

1. Preheat the oven to 350°F. Line a large baking sheet with parchment paper.

2. In a medium bowl, combine the almonds, olive oil, rosemary, and sea salt, tossing to coat.

3. Spread the coated almonds onto the prepared baking sheet in a single layer. Roast for 10 minutes, then stir the almonds. Roast for another 8 to 10 minutes, or until the almonds are golden brown but not burned.

4. Remove the almonds from the oven and let cool for 10 minutes, or until they're cool enough to touch.

SWAP IT: For a smoky flavor, add 1 teaspoon of smoked paprika and ¾ teaspoon of garlic powder. Or if you want a sweet and spicy combo, toss the almonds in 1 to 2 tablespoons of honey and ¼ to ½ teaspoon of cayenne pepper.

Lemon-Turmeric Date Bites

MAKES 16 bites **PREP TIME**: 10 minutes, plus 15 minutes to freeze

30 MINUTES OR LESS | DAIRY-FREE | GLUTEN-FREE | NO-COOK | VEGAN

These Lemon-Turmeric Date Bites are great to have in the refrigerator for a quick and easy snack. Just make sure you have a high-power food processor. For the best texture, use dates that are still soft and sticky. If your dates are a bit dried out, soak them in hot water for 10 minutes before using. Store these date bites in an airtight container for up to 2 weeks in the refrigerator or 3 months in the freezer.

1 cup raw cashews

1 cup Medjool dates, pitted

Zest of 1 large lemon

Juice of ½ large lemon (about 2 tablespoons)

1 teaspoon ground turmeric

¼ teaspoon vanilla extract

⅛ teaspoon salt

2 tablespoons unsweetened shredded coconut

1 tablespoon chia seeds

Per serving (1 bite):
Calories: 87; Total fat: 4g; Saturated fat: 1g; Cholesterol: 0mg; Sodium: 23mg; Carbohydrates: 14g; Fiber: 2g; Sugar: 10g; Protein: 2g

1. In a food processor, pulse the cashews until you get a sand-like texture. Add the dates, lemon zest, lemon juice, turmeric, vanilla, and salt. Pulse a few times until the mixture is well combined and slightly sticky. You may need to scrape down the sides with a rubber spatula periodically. If the mixture isn't coming together, add a little water, 1 teaspoon at a time. You should be able to easily form the mixture into balls. Add the shredded coconut and chia seeds. Pulse another 3 or 4 times, or until well combined.

2. Set out a 9-inch-square baking dish. Using a tablespoon, form the mixture into medium balls. You should get about 16. Place the balls in the baking dish and freeze for 15 minutes.

SWAP IT: If lemon isn't your thing, leave out the lemon and turmeric and add 1 to 2 tablespoons of unsweetened cocoa powder and a pinch of cinnamon for a chocolaty treat.

Raspberry-Almond Chia Pudding

SERVES 2 **PREP TIME**: 5 minutes, plus 4 hours to chill

5-INGREDIENT | DAIRY-FREE | GLUTEN-FREE | NO-COOK | VEGETARIAN

Despite their small size, chia seeds are rich in nutrients that are important for brain health, including omega-3 fatty acids and B vitamins. They're also an excellent source of calcium, magnesium, and manganese. When soaked in water or milk, chia seeds have a unique gelling ability that creates a thick, pudding-like consistency. These puddings are healthy enough to enjoy as a make-ahead breakfast or snack yet sweet enough for dessert.

1 cup raspberries, fresh or frozen

1 cup unsweetened almond milk or any unsweetened milk you like

1 tablespoon honey

1 teaspoon vanilla extract

3 tablespoons chia seeds

Per serving: Calories: 323; Total fat: 13g; Saturated fat: 1g; Cholesterol: 0mg; Sodium: 178mg; Carbohydrates: 47g; Fiber: 18g; Sugar: 24g; Protein: 8g

1. In a blender, combine the raspberries, almond milk, honey, and vanilla. Blend on medium speed until fully combined. Pour the mixture into two jars or small bowls.

2. Divide the chia seeds evenly between the two jars and stir well to combine. Seal the jars with tight-fitting lids and place them in the refrigerator for at least 4 hours, or ideally overnight.

SWAP IT: To add a little tartness, add 2 tablespoons of lemon juice to the mixture when blending. To make this recipe vegan, use maple syrup instead of honey.

Frozen Greek Yogurt Bites

MAKES 12 bites **PREP TIME**: 10 minutes, plus 2 hours to freeze

5-INGREDIENT | GLUTEN-FREE | NO-COOK | VEGETARIAN

Craving a cold sweet treat? These Frozen Greek Yogurt Bites are made with just three ingredients and require minimal prep work. The hardest part is being patient while they freeze. For the fruit, feel free to use blueberries, raspberries, or diced strawberries. You can also add a small splash of vanilla extract. These tasty treats will keep for up to 3 weeks in the freezer.

1 cup low-fat plain Greek yogurt

1 cup berries

2 tablespoons honey (optional)

Per serving (1 bite):
Calories: 22; Total fat: 0g; Saturated fat: 0g; Cholesterol: 2mg; Sodium: 8mg; Carbohydrates: 2g; Fiber: 0g; Sugar: 2g; Protein: 2g

1. In a blender or food processor, blend the yogurt, berries, and honey (if using) on medium speed until the mixture is smooth and creamy.

2. Using a small spoon or a piping bag, transfer the yogurt mixture to an ice cube tray or individual mini silicon cupcake liners. If you're using an ice cube tray, you should get approximately 12 Greek yogurt bites. If you're using mini cupcake liners, you'll end up with closer to 24 mini bites.

3. Place the ice cube tray or mini liners in the freezer and let the yogurt bites set for at least 2 hours. Transfer them to a freezer-safe bag or container for storage.

MAKE IT EASIER: Mash together the yogurt, fruit, and honey in a large bowl using the back of a spoon, instead of pulling out the blender. You'll have chunks of fruit in your bites, but they'll be just as tasty.

No-Bake Berry Fruit Pizza

SERVES 8 **PREP TIME**: 15 minutes, plus 15 minutes to freeze

30 MINUTES OR LESS | GLUTEN-FREE | NO-COOK | VEGETARIAN

When I was growing up, fruit pizza was one of my favorite desserts. My mom would make a large sugar cookie, spread it with cream cheese frosting, and add a variety of sliced fruits on top. This recipe is a no-bake, healthier twist on that childhood classic. Feel free to get creative with your fruit toppings. One of my favorite combinations is blueberries, sliced strawberries, and sliced kiwi. Leftovers will keep in the refrigerator for up to 3 days.

1½ cups packed Medjool dates, pitted

1½ cups raw cashews

¾ teaspoon vanilla extract, divided

⅛ teaspoon salt

1 cup low-fat plain Greek yogurt

½ tablespoon freshly squeezed lemon juice

Fresh fruit, sliced

Per serving (without the fruit): Calories: 277; Total fat: 11g; Saturated fat: 2g; Cholesterol: 3mg; Sodium: 51mg; Carbohydrates: 40g; Fiber: 4g; Sugar: 31g; Protein: 8g

1. In a food processor, combine the dates, cashews, ½ teaspoon of vanilla, and salt. Pulse several times until the ingredients are well combined and the mixture is sticky enough to hold together when pressed into a ball. If the mixture is too crumbly, add a little water, 1 teaspoon at a time.

2. Using a rubber spatula, transfer the mixture to a 9-inch tart pan or pie dish. Press the mixture evenly into the pan and place it in the freezer for 15 minutes to set.

3. In a small bowl, whisk together the Greek yogurt, the lemon juice, and the remaining ¼ teaspoon of vanilla extract. Taste and add more lemon juice as needed. Using a rubber spatula, evenly spread the Greek yogurt topping over the prepared crust.

4. Add any fruit you like on top of the yogurt topping. Serve immediately or chill in the freezer for 1 hour for a firmer yogurt topping.

SWAP IT: To make this recipe vegan, use a plant-based yogurt in place of the Greek yogurt. You can also adjust the flavor of the Greek yogurt topping by adding almond, orange, or lemon extract.

Avocado Chocolate Truffles

MAKES 12 truffles **PREP TIME**: 10 minutes, plus 30 minutes to chill
COOK TIME: 5 minutes

5-INGREDIENT | DAIRY-FREE | GLUTEN-FREE | ONE-POT | VEGAN

These truffles are rich, indulgent, and healthier than traditional chocolate truffles. For a more nutritious spin, they get their creamy consistency from mashed avocado rather than heavy cream and butter. To make them just as pretty as you'd buy them at the store, roll your truffles in a little unsweetened cocoa powder. Store leftover truffles in an airtight container for up to 3 days in the refrigerator.

6 ounces dark chocolate, chopped, vegan if needed

1 teaspoon vanilla extract

⅓ cup mashed avocado (about 1 small avocado)

Pinch salt

¼ cup unsweetened cocoa powder

Per serving (1 truffle):
Calories: 109; Total fat: 8g; Saturated fat: 4g; Cholesterol: 0mg; Sodium: 17mg; Carbohydrates: 9g; Fiber: 3g; Sugar: 4g; Protein: 2g

1. In a double boiler or a metal bowl set over a pot of boiling water, warm the chocolate and vanilla over medium-high heat, stirring frequently until the chocolate has fully melted, about 4 minutes.

2. Remove the chocolate from the stove and stir in the avocado and salt. Transfer the avocado mixture to the refrigerator and chill for 20 minutes, or until the mixture is slightly hardened.

3. Place the cocoa powder in a shallow bowl and set it aside. Line a baking sheet with parchment paper and set it next to the cocoa powder. Remove the avocado mixture from the refrigerator. Using a tablespoon, scoop out a portion and roll it into a small ball. Gently roll the ball in cocoa powder and place it on the prepared baking sheet. Repeat with the remaining mixture.

4. Place the rolled truffles in the refrigerator for 10 minutes to chill before enjoying.

SWAP IT: You can also coat some of the truffles in finely shredded coconut for a variation in taste, color, and texture.

Rustic Blueberry-Peach Crisp

SERVES 6 **PREP TIME**: 10 minutes / **COOK TIME**: 35 minutes

DAIRY-FREE | GLUTEN-FREE | ONE-PAN | VEGAN

Peach crisp is a classic summer dessert that's usually made with butter and is high in sugar. This version gets a MIND diet makeover by relying on the fruit itself for sweetness. It also uses heart-healthy avocado oil in place of the butter. Avocado oil has many of the same nutritional benefits as extra-virgin olive oil but has a milder flavor that works well in desserts. However, feel free to use olive oil if you don't have avocado oil on hand.

3 medium fresh peaches, pitted and sliced

1 cup blueberries, fresh or frozen

1 tablespoon freshly squeezed lemon juice

1 tablespoon cornstarch

1 cup old-fashioned rolled oats, gluten-free if needed

¼ cup slivered almonds

1 teaspoon cinnamon

½ teaspoon ground ginger

¼ teaspoon ground nutmeg

2 tablespoons avocado oil

1 tablespoon pure maple syrup

Per serving: Calories: 178; Total fat: 8g; Saturated fat: 1g; Cholesterol: 0mg; Sodium: 2mg; Carbohydrates: 25g; Fiber: 4g; Sugar: 11g; Protein: 4g

1. Preheat the oven to 350°F.

2. In a 10-inch tart pan or a 9-by-9-inch baking dish, mix together the peaches, blueberries, lemon juice, and cornstarch until well combined. Set aside.

3. In a medium bowl, combine the oats, almonds, cinnamon, ginger, nutmeg, oil, and maple syrup until well combined. Spread the topping over the filling in an even layer.

4. Bake for 30 to 35 minutes, or until the fruit juices are bubbling and the top is a light golden brown. Serve immediately.

SWAP IT: Swap out the peaches and blueberries with in-season fruits, such as apples or pears in the fall and strawberries and rhubarb in the spring.

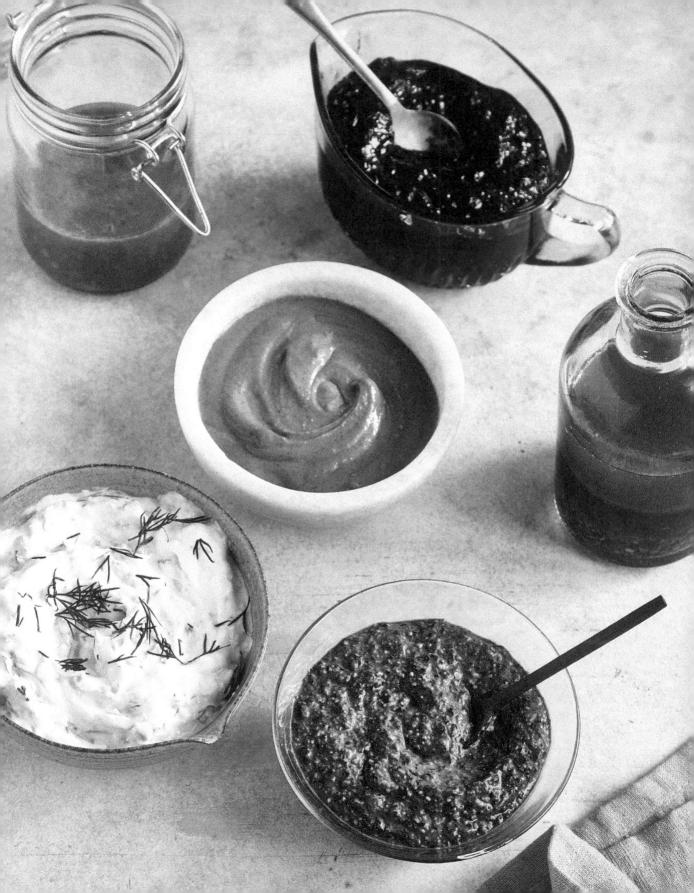

CHAPTER 9

Dressings and Sauces

Lemon-Dijon Dressing

MAKES about ½ cup **PREP TIME**: 5 minutes

30 MINUTES OR LESS | DAIRY-FREE | GLUTEN-FREE | NO-COOK | VEGAN

This Lemon-Dijon Dressing is the perfect go-to dressing. Not only is it made with ingredients you likely have on hand, but it also pairs with a wide variety of salad ingredients. Make a bigger batch so that you can use it throughout the week.

Zest of ½ medium lemon

2 tablespoons freshly squeezed lemon juice

½ teaspoon Dijon mustard

1 garlic clove, minced

¼ teaspoon salt

⅛ teaspoon freshly ground black pepper

¼ cup extra-virgin olive oil

**Per serving
(2 tablespoons):** Calories: 123; Total fat: 14g; Saturated fat: 2g; Cholesterol: 0mg; Sodium: 163mg; Carbohydrates: 1g; Fiber: 0g; Sugar: 0g; Protein: 0g

In a small bowl, whisk together the lemon zest, lemon juice, mustard, garlic, salt, and pepper. While continuing to whisk, slowly pour the olive oil into the mixture until fully combined.

SWAP IT: This dressing also works well with the zest and juice of other citrus fruits, including oranges, grapefruits, and limes. For extra flavor, add chopped fresh herbs, such as mint or thyme.

Five-Ingredient Ginger Dressing

MAKES about ¾ cup **PREP TIME**: 10 minutes

5-INGREDIENT | 30 MINUTES OR LESS | DAIRY-FREE | GLUTEN-FREE
NO-COOK | VEGAN

Inspired by a salad dressing from a local restaurant, this Five-Ingredient Ginger Dressing has a little kick from the fresh ginger that pairs well with the mild sweetness of the rice vinegar. The next time you make an Asian-inspired salad, skip the sugary bottled dressings from the store and use this homemade version instead. It will keep for up to 2 weeks in the refrigerator.

2 tablespoons grated fresh ginger

1 garlic clove, minced

2 tablespoons low-sodium soy sauce, gluten-free if needed

¼ cup rice vinegar

½ cup extra-virgin olive oil

**Per serving
(2 tablespoons):** Calories: 165; Total fat: 18g; Saturated fat: 3g; Cholesterol: 0mg; Sodium: 192mg; Carbohydrates: 2g; Fiber: 0g; Sugar: 1g; Protein: 1g

In a small bowl, whisk together the ginger, garlic, soy sauce, and vinegar. While continuing to whisk, slowly pour the olive oil into the dressing to combine.

SWAP IT: If you can't find gluten-free soy sauce, use low-sodium tamari or coconut aminos instead.

Three-Ingredient Blueberry Chia Seed Jam

MAKES 1 cup **PREP TIME**: 5 minutes, plus 10 minutes to set / **COOK TIME**: 15 minutes

5-INGREDIENT | 30 MINUTES OR LESS | DAIRY-FREE | GLUTEN-FREE
ONE-POT | VEGAN

While traditional jam recipes require pectin and large amounts of sugar to thicken, this three-ingredient jam uses the gelling properties of chia seeds to create an easier and healthier alternative. Sweetened with frozen blueberries and pure maple syrup, this jam goes perfectly with a stack of Oatmeal Blender Pancakes (page 40) or stirred into plain Greek yogurt. Use the jam immediately or allow it to cool completely before storing it in the refrigerator for up to 2 weeks.

1 pound frozen blueberries

2 tablespoons pure maple syrup

2 tablespoons chia seeds

Per serving (1 tablespoon):
Calories: 27; Total fat: 1g; Saturated fat: 0g; Cholesterol: 0mg; Sodium: 1mg; Carbohydrates: 6g; Fiber: 1g; Sugar: 4g; Protein: 0g

1. In a medium skillet over medium heat, combine the blueberries and maple syrup. Stir the mixture frequently until it comes to a low boil, about 10 minutes.

2. Using a potato masher or fork, carefully mash the blueberries. Continue to cook for 3 to 4 minutes. Stir in the chia seeds and cook for 1 more minute.

3. Remove the skillet from the heat and let the mixture sit for 10 minutes, or until thickened. Transfer the mixture to a jar.

SWAP IT: If you prefer strawberry jam, simply use 1 pound of frozen strawberries instead of the blueberries. You can also add 1 teaspoon of vanilla extract after cooking for a touch of vanilla flavor.

Family-Favorite Peanut Sauce

MAKES 1 cup **PREP TIME**: 10 minutes

30 MINUTES OR LESS | DAIRY-FREE | GLUTEN-FREE | NO-COOK | VEGAN

This recipe was passed down to me by a friend's family. I still remember the first time I tasted it, having that "aha" moment. Despite numerous attempts at making a peanut sauce, this was the first that had a clean peanut flavor that wasn't overly salty. Over the years, I've tweaked the recipe slightly, adding ground ginger and red pepper flakes for extra zing.

½ cup natural peanut butter, smooth or chunky

½ cup hot water

1 tablespoon low-sodium soy sauce, gluten-free if needed

1 teaspoon apple cider vinegar

1 teaspoon garlic powder

½ teaspoon ground ginger

Pinch red pepper flakes

**Per serving
(2 tablespoons):** Calories: 97; Total fat: 8g; Saturated fat: 1g; Cholesterol: 0mg; Sodium: 73mg; Carbohydrates: 4g; Fiber: 1g; Sugar: 1g; Protein: 4g

1. In a medium bowl, whisk together the peanut butter and hot water until smooth. Stir in the soy sauce, vinegar, garlic powder, and ginger.

2. Taste and adjust the garlic and ginger before adding red pepper flakes to taste. Let the mixture sit for 5 minutes to thicken before serving.

SWAP IT: I find using garlic powder and ground ginger results in a smoother texture. But you can sub in 2 teaspoons of minced fresh garlic and 2 tablespoons of grated fresh ginger.

Simple Tzatziki

MAKES 2½ cups **PREP TIME**: 15 minutes

30 MINUTES OR LESS | GLUTEN-FREE | NO-COOK | VEGETARIAN

Tzatziki is a traditional Greek sauce made with yogurt, cucumber, extra-virgin olive oil, lemon juice, garlic, and fresh herbs. Although you can enjoy it year-round, I especially like it In the summer because it's just so refreshing. For the most nutrients, don't peel your cucumber. Simply cut off the ends and grate the whole cucumber using a cheese grater. Serve immediately or store in an airtight container in the refrigerator for up to 4 days.

2 cups grated cucumber, squeezed and drained of excess liquid

1½ cups low-fat plain Greek yogurt

2 tablespoons extra-virgin olive oil

1 tablespoon freshly squeezed lemon juice

2 tablespoons chopped fresh dill

1 garlic clove, grated

¼ teaspoon salt

Per serving (¼ cup):
Calories: 57; Total fat: 4g; Saturated fat: 1g; Cholesterol: 3mg; Sodium: 73mg; Carbohydrates: 3g; Fiber: 0g; Sugar: 2g; Protein: 4g

In a large bowl, combine the cucumber, yogurt, olive oil, lemon juice, dill, garlic, and salt. Taste and adjust the seasonings as needed.

MAKE IT EASIER: Rather than grating the cucumber by hand, use the shredding blade on your food processor. After removing the cucumber, add the S-blade back into the food processor and add the remaining ingredients to make your sauce.

Fresh Herb Chimichurri

MAKES ½ cup **PREP TIME**: 10 minutes

30 MINUTES OR LESS │ DAIRY-FREE │ GLUTEN-FREE │ NO-COOK │ VEGAN

Chimichurri is a traditional Argentine sauce. Although it's typically made with parsley, this recipe adds an extra layer of flavor by also adding fresh cilantro. Chimichurri is often paired with red meat, but it goes just as well with firm white fish, poultry, and tofu. I recommend drizzling it on top of the Fish en Papillote with Summer Squash (page 99). Store leftovers in an airtight container in the refrigerator for up to 1 week.

1 small shallot, minced

1 garlic clove, minced

2 tablespoons extra-virgin olive oil

2 tablespoons apple cider vinegar

¼ teaspoon salt

2 tablespoons finely chopped fresh parsley

2 tablespoons chopped fresh cilantro

1 tablespoon water

⅛ teaspoon freshly ground black pepper

Per serving (1 tablespoon):
Calories: 282; Total fat: 27g; Saturated fat: 4g; Cholesterol: 0mg; Sodium: 602mg; Carbohydrates: 9g; Fiber: 2g; Sugar: 3g; Protein: 2g

1. In a small bowl, combine the shallot, garlic, olive oil, vinegar, and salt. Allow the mixture to sit for 5 minutes.

2. Stir in the parsley, cilantro, water, and pepper. Taste and adjust the seasonings as needed.

SWAP IT: If you don't like cilantro, you can use all parsley. You can also use mint in place of the cilantro for a Thai-inspired flavor.

Vegan Spinach Pesto

MAKES about 1 cup **PREP TIME**: 10 minutes

30 MINUTES OR LESS | DAIRY-FREE | GLUTEN-FREE | NO-COOK | VEGAN

This Vegan Spinach Pesto puts a MIND diet twist on more traditional pesto recipes by substituting some of the basil for fresh spinach and leaving out the Parmesan cheese. In addition to mixing it with pasta, this vegan pesto is delicious over grain bowls and cooked proteins like fish and chicken. Store leftovers in an airtight container in the refrigerator for up to 2 days.

½ cup pine nuts, toasted

2 tablespoons freshly squeezed lemon juice

1 garlic clove

¼ teaspoon salt

⅛ teaspoon freshly ground black pepper

2 cups fresh baby spinach

½ cup fresh basil

¼ cup extra-virgin olive oil

Per serving (2 tablespoons): Calories: 117; Total fat: 12g, Saturated fat: 2g; Cholesterol: 0mg; Sodium: 86mg; Carbohydrates: 2g; Fiber: 1g; Sugar: 1g; Protein: 1g

1. In a food processor, pulse the pine nuts, lemon juice, garlic, salt, and pepper until the pine nuts are chopped into small pieces. Add the spinach and basil. Pulse until the mixture is well combined.

2. With the food processor running on low, drizzle in the olive oil. Pulse to combine. Taste and adjust the salt and pepper, as needed.

SWAP IT: If you miss the cheesy flavor of traditional pesto, add nutritional yeast, 1 teaspoon at a time, until it tastes the way you like.

Hidden Veggie Marinara Sauce

MAKES 4 cups **PREP TIME**: 15 minutes / **COOK TIME**: 25 minutes

DAIRY-FREE | GLUTEN-FREE | ONE-POT | VEGAN

Store-bought tomato sauces are often high in salt and sugar. By making your own at home, you get full control over the ingredients going into your sauce. Plus, a homemade sauce tastes way better than something you'd pour from a jar! This Hidden Veggie Marinara Sauce will quickly become a family staple, as it's simple to make and is an easy way to add more vegetables into your meals. To store leftovers, allow the sauce to cool completely, then store it in an airtight container in the refrigerator for up to 5 days.

2 tablespoons
extra-virgin olive oil

½ cup grated onion

2 garlic cloves, grated

1 large carrot, grated

1 large zucchini, grated

1 cup finely chopped
mushrooms

1 (28-ounce) can
no-added-salt
tomato sauce

2 tablespoons
tomato paste

1 teaspoon Italian
seasoning

1 teaspoon salt

½ teaspoon freshly
ground black pepper

1 bay leaf (optional)

1. In a medium pot, heat the oil over medium-high heat. Add the onion, garlic, carrot, zucchini, and mushrooms. Sauté until the garlic is fragrant and the vegetables start to soften slightly, about 3 minutes.

2. Add the tomato sauce, tomato paste, Italian seasoning, salt, pepper, and bay leaf (if using). Bring the sauce to a boil, then reduce the heat to low and simmer for 20 minutes, stirring occasionally. Taste and adjust the seasonings, as needed.

SWAP IT: For even more vegetable goodness, add chopped kale or spinach into the sauce, as well. If you don't like mushrooms, chopped eggplant is a good alternative.

Per serving (½ cup):
Calories: 93; Total fat: 4g;
Saturated fat: 1g; Cholesterol: 0mg; Sodium: 332mg;
Carbohydrates: 13g; Fiber: 4g;
Sugar: 8g; Protein: 2g

BLANK MEAL PLAN

Visit CallistoMediaBooks.com/minddietforbeginners to download extra copies of the meal plan. You can also photocopy this page.

	BREAKFAST	LUNCH	DINNER
MON			
TUES			
WED			
THUR			
FRI			
SAT			
SUN			

MIND DIET FOOD TRACKER

This MIND Diet Food Tracker will help you track your adherence to the MIND diet each week without needing to follow a set meal plan. Simply make a tally mark in the corresponding food group box each time you eat something during the day. For example, if you have a smoothie with unsweetened almond milk, 1 cup of spinach, and 1 cup of blueberries, you'd put one tally mark in both the "berries" and "green leafy vegetables" boxes. Similarly, if you have 1 cup of ice cream, you'd put two tally marks in the "sweets" box, as 1 cup of ice cream is two servings.

Visit CallistoMediaBooks.com/minddietforbeginners to download extra copies of the food tracker. You can also photocopy page 149.

FOOD (RECOMMENDED WEEKLY AMOUNT)	MON	TUES	WED	THUR	FRI	SAT	SUN
Green leafy vegetables (6+ per week)							
Other vegetables (1+ per day)							
Nuts (5+ per week)							
Beans and legumes (3+ per week)							
Whole grains (3 per day)							
Berries (2+ per week)							
Poultry (2+ per week)							
Fish (1+ per week)							
Eggs (up to 4 per week)							
Red meat (4 or less per week)							
Butter and margarine (1 tablespoon or less per day)							
Cheese (1 or less per week)							
Sweets (4 or less per week)							
Fried and fast foods (1 or less per week)							

MEASUREMENT CONVERSIONS

Volume Equivalents	U.S. STANDARD	U.S. STANDARD (OUNCES)	METRIC (APPROXIMATE)
Liquid	2 tablespoons	1 fl. oz.	30 mL
	¼ cup	2 fl. oz.	60 mL
	½ cup	4 fl. oz.	120 mL
	1 cup	8 fl. oz.	240 mL
	1½ cups	12 fl. oz.	355 mL
	2 cups or 1 pint	16 fl. oz.	475 mL
	4 cups or 1 quart	32 fl. oz.	1 L
	1 gallon	128 fl. oz.	4 L
Dry	⅛ teaspoon	–	0.5 mL
	¼ teaspoon	–	1 mL
	½ teaspoon	–	2 mL
	¾ teaspoon	–	4 mL
	1 teaspoon	–	5 mL
	1 tablespoon	–	15 mL
	¼ cup	–	59 mL
	⅓ cup	–	79 mL
	½ cup	–	118 mL
	⅔ cup	–	156 mL
	¾ cup	–	177 mL
	1 cup	–	235 mL
	2 cups or 1 pint	–	475 mL
	3 cups	–	700 mL
	4 cups or 1 quart	–	1 L
	½ gallon	–	2 L
	1 gallon	–	4 L

Oven Temperatures

FAHRENHEIT	CELSIUS (APPROX)
250°F	120°C
300°F	150°C
325°F	165°C
350°F	180°C
375°F	190°C
400°F	200°C
425°F	220°C
450°F	230°C

Weight Equivalents

U.S. STANDARD	METRIC (APPROX)
½ ounce	15 g
1 ounce	30 g
2 ounces	60 g
4 ounces	115 g
8 ounces	225 g
12 ounces	340 g
16 ounces or 1 pound	455 g

RESOURCES

If you're interested in learning more about or participating in MIND diet research, visit Mind-Diet-Trial.org.

For more information and resources on brain function and cognitive health, check out these organizations:

- ▶ AARP.org/health/brain-health/global-council-on-brain-health

- ▶ Act.Alz.org

- ▶ AlzFdn.org

- ▶ Alzheimer's Association

- ▶ Alzheimer's Foundation of America

- ▶ Global Council on Brain Health

- ▶ Memory.UCSF.edu

- ▶ National Institute on Aging

- ▶ NIA.NIH.gov

- ▶ Weill Institute for Neurosciences Memory and Aging Center at the University of California San Francisco

REFERENCES

Agarwal P., Y. Wang, A. S. Buchman, T. M. Holland, D. A. Bennett, and M. C. Morris. 2018. "MIND Diet Associated with Reduced Incidence and Delayed Progression of Parkinsonism in Old Age." *The Journal of Nutrition, Health and Aging* 22(10): 1211–1215. doi:10.1007/s12603-018-1094-5

Akbaraly, Tasnime N., Eric J. Brunner, Jane E. Ferrie, Michael G. Marmot, Mika Kivimaki, and Archana Singh-Manoux. 2009. "Dietary Pattern and Depressive Symptoms in Middle Age." *British Journal of Psychiatry: The Journal of Mental Science* 195(5): 408–413. doi:10.1192/bjp.bp.108.058925

Amen, Daniel G., William S. Harris, Parris M. Kidd, Somayeh Meysami, and Cyrus A. Raji. 2017. "Quantitative Erythrocyte Omega-3 EPA plus DHA Levels Are Related to Higher Regional Cerebral Blood Flow on Brain SPECT." *Journal of Alzheimer's Disease: JAD* 58(4): 1189–1199. doi:10.3233/JAD-170281

Chen, Xi, Brooke Maguire, Henry Brodaty, and Fiona O'Leary. 2019. "Dietary Patterns and Cognitive Health in Older Adults: A Systematic Review." *Journal of Alzheimer's Disease: JAD* 67(2): 583–619. doi:10.3233/JAD-180468 [Published correction appears in *Journal of Alzheimer's Disease: JAD* 69(2): 595–596.]

Echouffo-Tcheugui, Justin B., Sarah C. Conner, Jayandra J. Himali, Pauline Maillard, Charles S. DeCarli, Alexa S. Beiser, Ramachandran S. Vasan, and Sudha Seshadri. 2018. "Circulating Cortisol and Cognitive and Structural Brain Measures: The Framingham Heart Study." *Neurology* 91(21): e1961–1970. doi:10.1212/WNL.0000000000006549

Edwards, George A., III, Nazaret Gamez, Gabriel Escobedo Jr, Olivia Calderon, and Ines Moreno-Gonzalez. 2019. "Modifiable Risk Factors for Alzheimer's Disease." *Frontiers in Aging Neuroscience* 11: 146. doi:10.3389/fnagi.2019.00146

Emory University. "Cognitive Skill and Normal Aging." alzheimers.Emory.edu/healthy_aging/cognitive-skills-normal-aging.html

Eugene, Andy R., and Jolanta Masiak. 2015. "The Neuroprotective Aspects of Sleep." *MEDtube Science* 3(1): 35–40.

Féart, Catherine, Cécilia Samieri, and Pascale Barberger-Gateau. 2010. "Mediterranean Diet and Cognitive Function in Older Adults." *Current Opinion in Clinical Nutrition and Metabolic Care* 13(1): 14–18. doi:10.1097/MCO.0b013e3283331fe4

Feng, Lei, Irwin Kee-Mun Cheah, Maisie Mei-Xi Ng, Jialiang Li, Sue Mei Chan, Su Lin Lim, Rathi Mahendran, Ee-Heok Kua, and Barry Halliwell. 2019. "The Association between Mushroom Consumption and Mild Cognitive Impairment:

A Community-Based Cross-Sectional Study in Singapore." *Journal of Alzheimer's Disease: JAD* 68(1): 197–203. doi:10.3233/JAD-180959

Gómez-Pinilla, Fernando. 2008. "Brain Foods: The Effects of Nutrients on Brain Function." *Nature Reviews. Neuroscience* 9(7): 568–78. doi:10.1038/nrn2421

Harada, Caroline N., Marissa C. Natelson Love, and Kristen L. Triebel. 2013. "Normal Cognitive Aging." *Clinics in Geriatric Medicine* 29(4): 737-752. doi:10.1016/j.cger.2013.07.002

Hosking, Diane E., Ranmalee Eramudugolla, Nicolas Cherbuin, and Kaarin J. Anstey. 2019. "MIND Not Mediterranean Diet Related to 12-Year Incidence of Cognitive Impairment in an Australian Longitudinal Cohort Study." *Alzheimer's & Dementia: The Journal of the Alzheimer's Association* 15(4): 581–89. doi:10.1016/j.jalz.2018.12.011

Karr, Justin E., Raquel B. Graham, Scott M. Hofer, and Graciela Muniz-Terrera. 2018. "When Does Cognitive Decline Begin? A Systematic Review of Change Point Studies on Accelerated Decline in Cognitive and Neurological Outcomes Preceding Mild Cognitive Impairment, Dementia, and Death." *Psychology and Aging* 33(2): 195–218. doi:10.1037/pag0000236

Kennedy, David O. 2016. "B Vitamins and the Brain: Mechanisms, Dose and Efficacy—A Review." *Nutrients* 8(2): 68. doi:10.3390/nu8020068

La Fata, Giorgio, Peter Weber, and M. Hasan Mohajeri. 2014. "Effects of Vitamin E on Cognitive Performance during Ageing and in Alzheimer's Disease." *Nutrients* 6(12): 5453–72. doi:10.3390/nu6125453

Melo, Helen M., Luís Eduardo Santos, and Sergio T. Ferreira. 2019. "Diet-Derived Fatty Acids, Brain Inflammation, and Mental Health." *Frontiers in Neuroscience* 13: 265. doi:10.3389/fnins.2019.00265

Morris, Martha Clare, Christy C. Tangney, Yamin Wang, Frank M. Sacks, David A. Bennett, and Neelum T. Aggarwal. 2015. "MIND Diet Associated with Reduced Incidence of Alzheimer's Disease." *Alzheimer's & Dementia: The Journal of the Alzheimer's Association* 11(9): 1007–14. doi:10.1016/j.jalz.2014.11.009

Morris, Martha Clare, Christy C. Tangney, Yamin Wang, Frank M. Sacks, Lisa L. Barnes, David A. Bennett, and Neelum T. Aggarwal. 2015. "MIND Diet Slows Cognitive Decline with Aging." *Alzheimer's & Dementia: The Journal of the Alzheimer's Association* 11(9): 1015–22. doi:10.1016/j.jalz.2015.04.011

National Institute on Aging. 2019. "Alzheimer's Disease Fact Sheet." NIA.NIH.gov/health/alzheimers-disease-fact-sheet

Nettleton, Jodi E., Teja Klancic, Alana Schick, Ashley C. Choo, Jane Shearer, Stephanie L. Borgland, Faye Chleilat, Shyamchand Mayengbam, and Raylene A. Reimer. 2019. "Low-Dose Stevia (Rebaudioside A) Consumption Perturbs Gut

Microbiota and the Mesolimbic Dopamine Reward System." *Nutrients* 11(6): 1248. doi:10.3390/nu11061248

Omar, Syed Haris. 2019. "Mediterranean and MIND Diets Containing Olive Bio-phenols Reduces the Prevalence of Alzheimer's Disease." *International Journal of Molecular Sciences* 20(11): 2797. doi:10.3390/ijms20112797

Pase, Matthew P., Jayandra J. Himali, Alexa S. Beiser, Hugo J. Aparicio, Claudia L. Satizabal, Ramachandran S. Vasan, Sudha Seshadri, and Paul F. Jacques. 2017. "Sugar- and Artificially Sweetened Beverages and the Risks of Incident Stroke and Dementia: A Prospective Cohort Study." *Stroke: A Journal of Cerebral Circulation* 48(5): 1139–46. doi:10.1161/STROKEAHA.116.016027

Poly, Coreyann, Joseph M. Massaro, Sudha Seshadri, Philip A. Wolf, Eunyoung Cho, Elizabeth Krall, Paul F. Jacques, and Rhoda Au. 2011. "The Relation of Dietary Choline to Cognitive Performance and White-Matter Hyperintensity in the Framingham Offspring Cohort." *The American Journal of Clinical Nutrition* 94(6): 1584–91. doi:10.3945/ajcn.110.008938

Rendeiro, Catarina, Justin S. Rhodes, and Jeremy P. E. Spencer. 2015. "The Mech-anisms of Action of Flavonoids in the Brain: Direct versus Indirect Effects." *Neurochemistry International* 89: 126–39. doi:10.1016/j.neuint.2015.08.002

Smith, A. David, Stephen M. Smith, Celeste A. de Jager, Philippa Whitbread, Carole Johnston, Grzegorz Agacinski, Abderrahim Oulhaj, Kevin M. Bradley, Robin Jacoby, and Helga Refsum. 2010. "Homocysteine-Lowering by B Vitamins Slows the Rate of Accelerated Brain Atrophy in Mild Cognitive Impairment: A Random-ized Controlled Trial." *PloS One* 5(9): e12244. DOI.org/10.1371/journal.pone.0012244

Spencer, Jeremy P. E. 2009. "Flavonoids and Brain Health: Multiple Effects Under-pinned by Common Mechanisms." *Genes & Nutrition* 4(4): 243–50. doi:10.1007/s12263-009-0136-3

Stanford Health Care. "Risk Factors for Dementia." StanfordHealthCare.org/medical-conditions/brain-and-nerves/dementia/risk-factors.html

Subash, Selvaraju, Musthafa Mohamed Essa, Samir Al-Adawi, Mushtaq A. Memon, Thamilarasan Manivasagam, and Mohammed Akbar. 2014. "Neuroprotective Effects of Berry Fruits on Neurodegenerative Diseases." *Neural Regeneration Research* 9 (16): 1557–66. doi:10.4103/1673-5374.139483

2018 Physical Activity Guidelines Advisory Committee. 2018. "2018 Physical Activ-ity Guidelines Advisory Committee Scientific Report." Washington, D.C.: U.S. Department of Health and Human Services.

World Health Organization. 2019. "Risk Reduction of Cognitive Decline and Dementia: WHO Guidelines." NCBI.nlm.nih.gov/books/NBK542796

INDEX

ABOUT THE AUTHOR

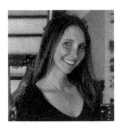 Kelli McGrane, MS, RD, is a registered dietitian based in Colorado. She has worked in inpatient and outpatient nutrition counseling at hospitals in Boston and in nutrition research for the University of Colorado. Currently, Kelli operates her own business, Kelli McGrane Nutrition LLC, where she provides evidence-based nutrition content, recipe development, and food photography for health-focused brands. She's been featured in major media outlets, including *Self*, *Women's Health*, *The Washington Post*, *CNN*, and *USA TODAY*.

When she isn't cooking or writing, you can find her in the mountains with her family and mini-Aussiedoodle, Bernie. For more of Kelli's work, visit TheHealthyToast.com or follow her on Instagram @thehealthytoast_rd.